Conventional Medicine

Alternative Medicine

Caroline Green

Consulting Editors
Beverly Green, M.D.
Christopher Ryan, M.D.

Mosby

Mosby is an imprint of Mosby—Year Book, Inc.

Published in the United States by
Mosby—Year Book, Inc.
11830 Westline Industrial Drive
St. Louis, MO 63146

ISBN: 0-916363-17-1 First Edition

Project Editor Marion Fisher
Project Art Editor Helen Spencer
Managing Editor Lindsay McTeague
Editorial Director Sophie Collins
Art Director Sean Keogh
Production Nikki Ingram
Developmental Editors
   David Manhoff, Cary Barbor

The publishers wish to thank Dr. Penny Stanway
for reviewing this book.

Note: The terms "he" and "she," used in
alternate sections, refer to people of both sexes,
unless a topic or sequence of photographs applies
only to a male or female.

Printed in Hong Kong

Biographical information

Beverly Green, M.D.
Dr. Green is Board Certified in Family Medicine
with a masters degree in Public Health. She
received her M.D. at the Medical College of Ohio,
and was a Robert Wood Johnson Fellow and
Preventive Medicine Resident at the University of
Washington. She is currently a Family Physician
in Poulsbo, WA, as well as a Clinical Instructor at
the UW Medical School.

Christopher Ryan, M.D.
Dr. Ryan is a graduate of Boston University
School of Medicine. He is on the staff of both the
Deaconess-Waltham and The Newton-Wellesley
Hospitals, and practices in West Newton, MA. Dr.
Ryan is Board Certified in both Family Medicine
and Geriatrics, and pursues post-graduate work at
The New England School of Homeopathy. He has
made use of nutritional and lifestyle modification
to help support healing and prevent disease since
the beginning of his practice, in combination with
conventional Western medicine, where appropriate.

Preface

This book is intended to provide general
information concerning medical conditions. It is
not intended to replace consultation with your
doctor or healthcare professional. Many hours
have been spent checking and rechecking the
medicines, treatment and procedures to assure
accuracy. Unfortunately, some changes in medical
treatment do occur. Please consult your doctor or
health care professional if you have any questions.

Notice

The author and publisher of this book have taken
care to make certain that all medical techniques
and references are correct, and compatible with
national standards generally accepted at the time
of publication. The author and publisher disclaim
any liability, loss, injury, or damage incurred as a
consequence, directly ot indirectly, of the use and
application of the contents of this book.

INDEX

USING THE FACTFILE

This book is divided into six chapters: 1 Head & Chest Ailments; 2 Digestive Problems; 3 Aches & Pains; 4 Skin & Hair Problems; 5 Women's & Children's Health; and 6 Emotional Conditions, which is followed by a section on Alternative Health. If you know which subject you wish to look up, turn to the relevant tab. On each you will find a table of contents for that part of the book. If you are unsure where to find the information you need, turn to the alphabetical index on page 3.

Illustration
Drawings of medical conditions and photography illustrating alternative treatments can be found throughout the book.

Text
The text is clearly divided into a description of the problem, its causes, and what a medical doctor might do to treat it.

Tab
Color-coded subject dividers enable you to turn quickly to the section you need. Each divider offers a list of the subjects on pages that bear the same colored band.

When to see a doctor
Each subject has a box advising when an ailment requires medical attention. Extreme cases are given in **Warning!** boxes.

Symptoms
Each subject has a box outlining the significant symptoms of the illness.

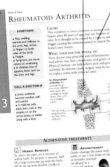

Alternative treatments
For each subject, alternative treatments are given to help relieve any symptoms.

Special features
Subjects of related interest appear in colored boxes on the relevant spread.

GENERAL INTRODUCTION

It can be troubling when you or a member of your family becomes ill, even if the illness is only minor. This book is intended to help you learn what steps to take to treat the most common medical problems. It will help you determine what actions to take when an illness does occur—whether it will be treatment at home, a visit to the doctor's office, or an emergency that requires calling an ambulance.

The symptoms given will help you identify the illness, and the causes will explain what may have triggered it. In some cases, removing the cause may be enough to get rid of the symptoms. You'll also find explanations of what type of treatment you should expect from a doctor, and there are recommendations on what symptoms should always be seen by a doctor. If in doubt, however, you should call your doctor's office for advice.

This book also provides alternative treatments, such as herbal remedies, homeopathy, and acupressure, that can be followed alongside your doctor's own advice. These are often intended to treat the symptoms and make you feel more comfortable; they are not recommended to replace your doctor's advice or treatment.

CHOOSING A PRACTITIONER

CALL A DOCTOR IF

- There is an unusual discharge or bleeding
- There is a marked change in your bowel or bladder habits
- A sore doesn't heal in 3 weeks
- A mole, freckle, or blemish changes color
- A lump appears in your breast
- You have a nagging cough or hoarseness
- You have chronic indigestion or difficulty in swallowing
- You experience sudden loss of weight or appetite
- You have recurrent vomiting
- There is unexplained severe pain, especially in the head, chest, or abdomen
- You have a high fever above 103°F (40°C)
- You have unexplained fainting or dizziness
- You have blurred vision or see a halo around lights
- You have severe shortness of breath
- Your lips, eyelids, or nails have a bluish tint
- Your ankles are severely swollen
- You have excessive thirst
- You have unusual weakness or fatigue
- There is yellowing of the skin or eyes
- As a man, you urinate often or with difficulty

FINDING A DOCTOR

If you do not already have a doctor, the best time to find one is when you are in good health. You will have the time to make a careful choice, and it will be easier for a doctor to assess your health.

Ask your friends and neighbors for a recommendation. Once you have a name, contact the doctor's office and ask for references, which will tell you about the doctor's professional qualifications.

Before and after your first visit, ask yourself the following questions:
- Is the doctor the age and gender that you feel most comfortable with?
- Is the office easy to travel to?
- Can you get an appointment without much delay?
- Is the office clean and are the staff courteous?
- Did you have to wait long to see the doctor?
- Did the doctor or health care provider put you at ease, listen to your main concerns, and answer the questions you had?
- If you were given a test or treatment (including medicine), did you understand what it was for, how to use it correctly, and what to do if you had a problem or a concern?
- Did you feel satisfied with your visit with the doctor or health care provider?

HOW CAN I GET THE BEST FROM MY DOCTOR?

Make sure you describe exactly what the problem is at the appointment. Don't expect the doctor to guess, and don't be afraid to ask questions. Make a note of things you would like to ask before your visit and take it along as a reminder.

If you don't think your doctor listens to you properly, or answers your questions as clearly as you would like, tell him so. If communication doesn't improve, however, you may want to change doctors.

In these situations you should seek a second opinion:
- Your doctor recommends surgery
- A rare or fatal disorder is diagnosed
- Your doctor does not make a diagnosis after several visits or tests and symptoms persist.

CHOOSING AN ALTERNATIVE PRACTITIONER

Always see your own doctor before consulting an alternative practitioner for a health problem. Make sure the practitioner is appropriately qualified by contacting the professional body for the particular therapy. Otherwise, ask the same questions that you would ask your regular doctor.

Head & Chest Ailments

HEAD & CHEST AILMENTS

You can experience many different illnesses in the upper part of your body. Ailments with symptoms that are usually specific to the head, apart from headache and migraine themselves, of course, include toothache, earache, infections of the eye and mouth, and a stuffy nose.

A temporary infection, such as a cold or flu, can start off as a runny nose but may spread to the throat, where it can cause tonsillitis, or down to the lungs, which can lead to bronchitis.

For many of these ailments, your doctor cannot prescribe pills to cure you. He may, however, suggest rest and over-the-counter drugs that will relieve the symptoms. Many alternative treatments can also be of great help.

Some people are affected by chronic conditions, such as asthma, which are beyond the scope of this book and should be treated in conjunction with a professional.

HEADACHES

SYMPTOMS

TENSION HEADACHE:
- A dull, steady pain
- Neck muscles may feel knotted
- Pain may be brief or long-lasting

MIGRAINE:
- Severe, usually one-sided throbbing pain
- Nausea
- Visual disturbances

CLUSTER HEADACHE:
- A mild aching feeling may precede an attack
- Severe pain around one eye, which may be red and watery
- Can occur several times a day for several weeks or months, with each one lasting from 30 minutes to 2 hours

SINUS HEADACHE:
- Pain behind the nose or in the forehead

CAUSES

- **Tension headaches** are caused by tightening of the muscles in the scalp, face, and neck due to stress or poor posture.
- **Migraines** result from the constriction and dilation of blood vessels caused by a chemical imbalance with many possible triggers.
- **Cluster headaches** occur mainly in men and are caused by a chemical imbalance in the brain.
- **Sinus headaches** are caused by inflammation and infection of the sinuses or when nasal congestion partially blocks a sinus. ▶

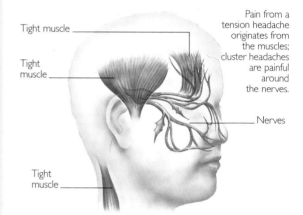

Tight muscle

Tight muscle

Tight muscle

Pain from a tension headache originates from the muscles; cluster headaches are painful around the nerves.

Nerves

ALTERNATIVE TREATMENTS

ACUPRESSURE
- You can relieve a headache by lightly pressing your middle finger between your eyebrows at the top of the bridge of your nose for 2 minutes.
- To relieve a tension headache, place the tips of your middle fingers in the hollows at the base of the skull on either side of the spine and press firmly for 1 minute.
- For a sinus headache in the forehead, place the tip of one finger in the bony notch a third of the way down the eyebrow from the nose. Press for 1 minute; release; and repeat 3 times.

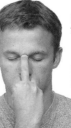

Pressure point between the eyebrows

HERBAL REMEDIES
For migraine take 3 125-mg capsules of feverfew leaf every 4 hours as needed. **Warning!** Do not take feverfew if pregnant.

WHAT YOUR DOCTOR WOULD DO

- Your doctor might suggest over-the-counter painkillers for a tension headache. You can also ask your pharmacist for advice on what to take.
- Your doctor may suggest you avoid loud noises and bright lights.
- For sinus headaches, your doctor may also recommend a decongestant.
- Rest and relaxation will benefit those with tension or sinus headaches, as will applying alternately hot and cold compresses.
- For migraines, your doctor may recommend one of a variety of drugs, in the form of pills or injections, depending on the frequency and severity of the attacks.
- If you suffer from migraines, your doctor may advise you to stop taking the contraceptive Pill and to avoid any foods and beverages, such as red wine, cheese, and chocolate, that trigger attacks.
- Relief from cluster headaches may require the prescription of a corticosteroid or other drug.
- Your doctor might take your blood pressure, suggest a vision test, and if concerned about other potentially serious causes of headache, might refer you to a specialist.

CALL A DOCTOR IF

- You have unusual or persistent headaches
- You have had a head injury and are drowsy, dizzy, nauseous, or have vomited

Warning!
Get medical help immediately if a headache is accompanied by: vomiting; high fever; limb weakness; double vision; slurred speech; a rash that does not fade when you press against it; a stiff neck.

 ### AROMATHERAPY
For a tension headache or migraine, blend a few drops of lavender oil into 2 teaspoons of sunflower oil and massage into the temples. For a sinus headache, eucalyptus may work better than lavender.

HOMEOPATHY
- For a sinus headache accompanied by mucus, try *Kali bichromicum* 6 or 12c, 2 pellets every 2 hours, for up to 4 doses (if no effect), or as needed for up to 2 days, if effective.

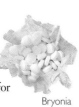
Bryonia

- For a headache aggravated by motion, try *Bryonia alba*. Take 30c 2 pellets every 30 minutes up to 4 times, then again every 4 hours up to 2 days if effective.

 ### REFLEXOLOGY
For a tension headache, press the thumb into the base of the big toe. Release after a few moments.

Reflexology point on the base of the big toe

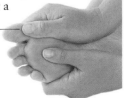

EARACHE

SYMPTOMS

INFECTION OF THE MIDDLE EAR:
- An aching or sharp pain inside the ear
- Fever
- Slight loss of hearing
- Discharge if the eardrum bursts

INFECTION OF THE EAR CANAL:
- Irritation or itching
- A discharge
- Mild deafness

EXCESS WAX:
- Sensation of fullness
- Partial deafness
- Irritated skin in ear canal

CAUSES

- An infection of the middle ear is the most common cause of earache in children.
- Middle-ear infections can result in a burst eardrum and a discharge from the ear. This relieves the pain because there is not as much pressure on the eardrum, but you should still see a doctor.
- If you swim often, bacteria may cause an infection of the ear canal (sometimes called swimmer's ear).
- Excess earwax in the ear canal doesn't hurt but can be irritating. ▶

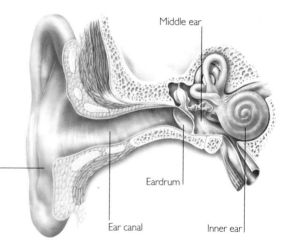

Middle ear

The pinna (the part that protrudes from the head) and ear canal are both parts of the outer ear.

Eardrum

Ear canal

Inner ear

ALTERNATIVE TREATMENTS

AROMATHERAPY

If the infection accompanies a cold, the cold should also be treated.

For a middle-ear infection, apply a hot compress soaked in a combination of chamomile and lavender essential oils floating on hot water to ease the pain.

To make the compress, sprinkle 4 or 5 drops of each of the essential oils into a bowl of hot water that is not so hot as to cause burning when touched. Fold a clean face cloth, handkerchief, or piece of towel or sheet and dip it into the bowl. Pick up as much of the oil floating on the surface as you can with the cloth. Wring out the compress before applying

it to the opening of the ear. Alternatively, you can massage the essential oils around the painful ear.

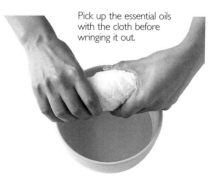

Pick up the essential oils with the cloth before wringing it out.

WHAT YOUR DOCTOR WOULD DO

Your doctor will look inside the ear for an infection, using an otoscope, a special instrument that has a light on the end, and will also examine the throat.

If there is infection in the middle ear, your doctor will probably prescribe antibiotics.

To ease the pain of an earache you can try placing a heating pad on the area, or you can use over-the-counter anesthetic ear drops. Over-the-counter pain relievers such as acetaminophen or ibuprofen can also decrease pain.

Excess wax can usually be painlessly removed at home using commercial preparations. Or, twice daily, for three days, place a few drops of warm mineral or baby oil in the ear. Then flush out the wax with a little warm water, using a bulb syringe. You should do this over a sink, after placing a towel over your shoulder to protect your clothing. If you notice no improvement after three days, consult your doctor, who will use a larger syringe to flush out the wax. Because of the amount of water involved, this can be a messy process, but it is usually completely painless.

CALL A DOCTOR IF

- The pain is severe
- You have a high fever
- There is a discharge from the ear
- There is sudden or prolonged deafness

Warning!

Never insert any object in your ear, including cotton swabs: they can puncture the fragile eardrum. If an object is lodged in your ear, you should have it removed by a doctor.

HOMEOPATHY

Homeopathic remedies can be used to treat the earache itself. But if the earache accompanies a cold, then the cold should be treated too.

- If the symptoms come on suddenly, after a chill, or exposure to cold dry wind, try *Aconite* 30c 2 pellets under the tongue every half hour up to 4 doses.
- If the onset is sudden, with a dramatic high fever, red face, hot dry head and cooler hands and feet, consider *Belladonna*, taken the same way.
- If there is creamy, yellow-green mucus from the nose and/or eye on the same side as the earache, and the patient is clingy, without thirst, and wants most to be held and comforted, try *Pulsatilla*, again, taken as above.

HERBAL REMEDIES

To soothe an inflamed ear canal, place 1–3 drops of warm mullein or garlic oil in it every 3 hours.
Warning! First, ask your doctor to make sure your eardrum is not perforated.

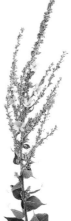

Verbascum thapsus, source of mullein oil

CONJUNCTIVITIS

SYMPTOMS

- Pain, irritation, and a gritty sensation in eye
- Redness and inflammation of eye

BACTERIAL CONJUNCTIVITIS:
- Green or yellow discharge

VIRAL CONJUNCTIVITIS:
- Increased tears

ALLERGY-RELATED CONJUNCTIVITIS:
- Itching, and swelling of the eyelid

CALL A DOCTOR IF

- The eye symptoms have not improved after 24 hours

CAUSES
- Bacteria, especially in children.
- Viruses that cause colds, sore throats, or measles.
- Irritants, including chlorine in swimming pools, smoke, dust, and allergens in cosmetics, pollen and animal hairs.

WHAT YOUR DOCTOR WOULD DO
For suspected bacterial conjunctivitis, your doctor will prescribe eye drops containing an antibiotic. For a young baby your doctor may take a swab to identify the infection. Conjunctivitis caused by a virus will disappear on its own. If an allergy has caused the problem, you'll be given eye drops containing an antihistamine or an anti-inflammatory drug.

Conjunctivitis, also called pinkeye, is an inflammation of the conjunctiva—the surface of the white of the eye.

Red, swollen eyelids   Inflamed eye white

ALTERNATIVE TREATMENTS

 HERBAL REMEDIES

Try an eyebath. Put 1 teaspoon of dried eyebright or 2–3 teaspoons of dried chamomile flowers into 1 pint (500 ml) of boiling water. Simmer for 15 minutes and strain. Let it cool. Apply it to the eye with a clean piece of cotton gauze 3 or 4 times a day, or use an eyecup to rinse the eye itself.

HOMEOPATHY
- Try *Pulsatilla* 6 or 12c 2 pellets every 2 hours as needed up to 2 days for a creamy yellow discharge, when the eye feels worse from wiping with a warm cloth, but is soothed by a cool one.
- *Apis* 6 or 12c as above may be helpful if the eye is swollen virtually shut.
- *Argentum nitricum* 6 or 12c as above may help bloodshot eyes that feel gritty and rough.

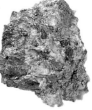

Argentum nitricum comes from the mineral silver nitrate.

STYES

SYMPTOMS

- Painful eyelid
- Redness and swelling
- Increased tears
- Sensitivity to bright lights

OUTSIDE THE LID:
- After several days it will burst, then heal

INSIDE THE LID:
- A fluid-filled cyst can persist

CALL A DOCTOR IF

- The stye does not improve within a few weeks
- It interferes with your vision
- Styes recur often

CAUSE
- A type of bacteria.

WHAT YOUR DOCTOR WOULD DO

Styes often disappear after a few days and don't require medical treatment. A warm compress relieves the soreness and inflammation, and may help the stye burst. With your eye closed, apply the compress 4 times daily for 10 to 15 minutes at a time.

If styes occur frequently, your doctor may prescribe antibiotics. A cyst from an internal stye may have to be removed by a doctor.

A stye is a small, pus-filled abscess near the edge of an eyelid. It usually develops on the outside of the eyelid but sometimes forms on the inside.

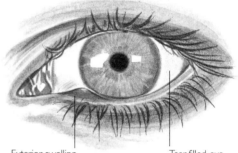

Exterior swelling   Tear-filled eye

ALTERNATIVE TREATMENTS

HERBAL REMEDIES
Eyedrops containing eyebright, made by a qualified herbal medicine practitioner, can help relieve the pain and inflammation.

HOMEOPATHY
If the usual warm cloth feels worse, but a cool one soothes, and the patient is affectionate and in need of hugs, try *Pulsatilla* 30c 2 pellets every hour for up to 6 doses.

Juice from the whole *Pulsatilla* plant is used.

OBJECT IN THE EYE

Try dislodging an object in the eye by blinking. If it won't budge, flush it out with clean filtered or bottled water. If it is still in the eye, gently lift the object out with a moistened tissue. To see the object, you can lift up your eyelid by gently grasping the lashes, but first wash your hands.
Warning! If the object is difficult to remove, call a doctor immediately. Do not try to remove anything embedded in the surface of the eye or resting on the iris (the colored part of the eye). Such an object must be removed by a doctor, usually under local anesthetic.

TOOTHACHE & GINGIVITIS

SYMPTOMS

TOOTHACHE:
- A dull throbbing pain
- Sharp stabbing pain, which may be worse when lying down
- Pain when biting or chewing
- Pain when the tooth is exposed to hot or cold temperatures

GINGIVITIS:
- Bleeding gums after brushing the teeth
- Red, swollen gums

CALL A DENTIST IF

- You have a sharp or throbbing pain
- A tooth is sensitive to heat or cold
- Gums are red, swollen, and painful

CAUSES
- A toothache is usually the result of tooth decay, although sometimes it is caused by a fractured tooth. Pain in the upper teeth may also be caused by a sinus infection.
- Gingivitis occurs when plaque (a sticky deposit made of food particles, bacteria, and mucus) builds up around the base of the teeth.

WHAT YOUR DENTIST WOULD DO
Painkillers help temporarily, but you must see a dentist for any toothache. Mild tooth decay requires a filling; more advanced decay or a broken tooth may need root canal treatment, in which the pulp—the living tissue of the tooth—is removed to save the tooth.

Your dentist will treat gingivitis by cleaning the teeth. If the mouth is sore, gargling with a pain-relieving mouthwash may be recommended. An antibiotic is prescribed if there is an infection. You can avoid gingivitis by brushing and flossing your teeth daily, avoiding snacks containing sugar or other refined carbohydrates between meals, and having regular dental checkups. If left untreated, gingivitis can lead to more serious gum diseases that can result in tooth loss.

ALTERNATIVE TREATMENTS

 HERBAL REMEDIES
Clove or myrrh oil rubbed directly on the gum around the painful tooth or onto sore gums can help relieve pain. **Warning!** Don't use these oils if pregnant.

ACUPRESSURE
To relieve the pain of a toothache, apply pressure to the depression to the side of the ankle bone on the inside of either leg for up to a minute. **Warning!** Do not do this if you are pregnant. It can bring on labor.

Acupressure point near the ankle bone

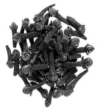

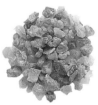

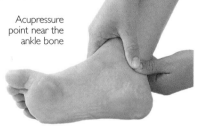

The flower buds and oil of cloves, a familiar spice, used in herbal remedies.

Myrrh is a resin from trees of the genus *Commiphora*.

COLD SORES & CANKER SORES

SYMPTOMS

COLD SORES:
- Small, red, painful blisters around the lips
- A burning or tingling sensation up to 24 hours before the sores appear

CANKER SORES:
- Small, painful, white or yellowish sores that last 5–10 days

CALL A DOCTOR IF

- A cold sore in the mouth doesn't go away after a 7–10 days
- A cold sore develops near an eye
- Canker sores are recurrent

Cold sores are small blisters that are usually found around the mouth, but they can occur on other parts of the body. Canker sores are painful ulcers that develop inside the mouth.

CAUSES
- Cold sores are caused by viruses including the *Herpes simplex* virus. Some people have an outbreak once; others have them repeatedly. Stress, colds, menstruation, and tiredness can trigger an outbreak.
- Canker sores occur more often in adolescents and in women before their monthly menstruation. They may be triggered by stress, allergy, or sunburns.

WHAT YOUR DOCTOR WOULD DO
There is no permanent cure for cold sores, but cream from a pharmacy reduces the pain. The doctor may prescribe an antiviral drug to help them heal faster. The virus is highly contagious. To avoid spreading it on yourself or to others, don't touch a sore. If you accidentally do, wash your hands immediately. Don't kiss anyone when you have a cold sore, and don't share towels or razors.

Canker sores can be healed with antiseptic mouthwashes. Or, mix one tablespoon of hydrogen peroxide with 8 oz (250 ml) of water. Swish it around in your mouth for several seconds and spit it out. Over-the-counter medicines also help relieve pain.

ALTERNATIVE TREATMENTS

AROMATHERAPY
To relieve either cold sores or canker sores, apply tea tree essential oil to the affected area, using a cotton swab.

REFLEXOLOGY
For a cold sore, press the top of the big toe, the face reflexology point, for one minute. Then apply pressure in the same position on the other toes, which relate to the teeth.

Reflexology point at top of big toe, just below the nail

VISUALIZATION
To reduce stress, close your eyes and for 15 minutes imagine yourself in a peaceful place, such as on a deserted beach or in the woods by a waterfall. Lying down helps, but you can also do this in a sitting position.

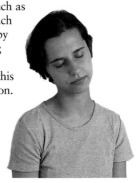

Listening to a tape of natural sounds can help you relax during visualization.

Hay Fever (allergic rhinitis)

SYMPTOMS

- A stuffy, runny nose
- Sneezing
- Headache
- Sore, watery, red eyes

CALL A DOCTOR IF

- You are uncertain which over-the-counter remedy to take
- Your symptoms worsen for no apparent reason

Sometimes certain substances trigger an exaggerated response in the immune system, causing the lining of the nose to become inflamed. Hay fever—allergy to fall seasonal pollen—is just one type of allergic rhinitis.

Causes

- Airborne pollen from flowers, grass, and trees causes hay fever.
- Other types of allergic rhinitis are caused by certain substances such as animal hair, feathers, house dust mites, air pollution, and chemicals in hairspray or perfume.

What your doctor would do

The best course of action is to avoid the allergy trigger, although this is not always possible. Feather-free pillows and hypoallergenic cosmetics are available, as are vacuum cleaners with special filtration systems to remove the house dust mites, which are common in most modern homes.

Over-the-counter antihistamine eye drops may provide relief. Because prolonged use of some nasal sprays and drops available from a pharmacy can damage the lining of the nose, seek advice from your doctor if your symptoms persist.

Alternative treatments

Aromatherapy

Inhaling the steam from 1 pint (500 ml) of very hot water containing a few drops of eucalyptus and peppermint oils eases sore sinuses. Or, mix a few drops of lavender in a base of almond oil and massage as shown.

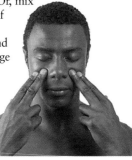

Massage nose, cheeks, and forehead with a few drops of lavender oil in almond oil.

Homeopathy

Allium cepa (red onion) 6 or 12c every hour or two as needed may be helpful where the eyes water freely and the runny nose burns the skin over the upper lip.

Acupressure

- Press the web of skin between the thumb and index finger for one minute.
Warning! Do not do this if you are pregnant.

Acupressure point at the web of the hand.

SINUSITIS

SYMPTOMS

- Pain and pressure in the forehead, bridge of the nose, and the cheekbones
- Sore, stuffy nose
- Thick nasal discharge

CALL A DOCTOR IF

- Symptoms do not improve in 7 days or if they recur more than 3 times in a year
- You develop an eye inflammation

Sinusitis is an inflammation or infection of the membranes lining the sinuses, which are the air-filled spaces in the bones surrounding the nose.

CAUSES
- Colds can cause swelling of the nasal membranes, and lead to sinusitis.
- Hay fever and other allergies can also cause swelling, obstructing one or more sinuses, leading to infection.

WHAT YOUR DOCTOR WOULD DO
Your doctor will probably recommend antibiotics, decongestants, and steam inhalations. In severe cases, or when sinusitis recurs frequently, you may need to have surgery to improve drainage in the sinuses.

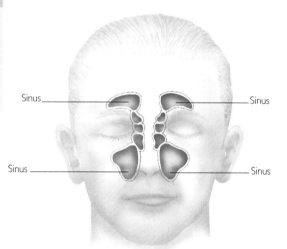

Sinus — — — Sinus

Sinus — — — Sinus

ALTERNATIVE TREATMENTS

 HERBAL REMEDIES
- Try taking 2 bromelain capsules by mouth 3 times daily on an empty stomach. This can have a remarkable mucus-thinning effect, easing the symptoms of sinusitis.

REFLEXOLOGY
Apply pressure to the top and sides of the toes.

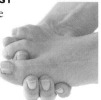

Reflexology points are at the top and sides of the toes.

NOSEBLEEDS

Nosebleeds are caused by a blow to the nose, fragile blood vessels, or removing encrusted material after a cold. To stop a nosebleed, sit up and lean slightly forward with your mouth open—this keeps blood from blocking the airways. Pinch the top of your nostrils and breathe through your mouth for 10 minutes. Release the nostrils slowly; do not blow your nose for 24 hours. If the bleeding doesn't stop after 20 minutes, call your doctor. **Warning!** If the nosebleed follows a blow to the head, get medical help immediately.

COLDS & FLU

SYMPTOMS

COLD:
- Blocked nose
- Headache
- Sore throat
- Watery eyes
- Cough—tickly, dry, or phlegmy

FLU:
- Any or all of the above, plus:
- Aching muscles and joints
- High fever

Almost everyone has experienced both the common cold and influenza, or flu. The problem is that it is often difficult to know if you have a bad cold or the flu. The simple answer is that you'll feel much worse if you have the flu.

CAUSES
Both colds and the flu are contagious viral infections that attack the air passages; the flu attacks other parts of the body, too. You can catch either by breathing in virus-infected air—in other words, being near an infected person who has just sneezed or coughed—or simply by shaking hands with them.

You do not catch a cold from being caught in the rain, going outside without a hat on, or sitting in a draft. Colds are most common in winter because people tend to spend more time indoors in close contact with each other and breathing hot dry air. Children seem to be more susceptible to colds partly because viruses are easily passed around crowded classrooms and partly because they have not yet built up the resistance to the many cold viruses that adults develop. Overall immune health, affected by stress and nutrition, is the key factor in not getting colds in the first place.

ALTERNATIVE TREATMENTS

HOMEOPATHY
- *Allium cepa* and *Nux vomica* are good for colds: take 6c every 4 hours for up to 10 doses.

Nux vomica

HERBAL REMEDIES
- Echinacea, osha, and lomatium are all effective immune stimulants. The best way to take them is as a fluid extract. Fill a dropper with the herbal remedy and mix it with a few ounces of water (or, squirt it directly into the throat) every few hours for the first 3–5 days of a cold or flu, continuing if necessary for

up to 2–3 weeks. (Using tonic herbs over a long period of time is not recommended. Always consult a trained herbalist if in doubt.)

ACUPRESSURE
To relieve coughing, bend your left elbow and make a fist, then place your right thumb on the crease of the elbow. Press firmly for 1 minute and repeat on the other arm. Do this 3 times.

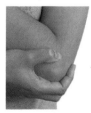

Point near elbow

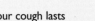

WHAT YOUR DOCTOR WOULD DO

Once you become ill, there are no drugs that will cure a cold or the flu—you'll have to let the disease run its course. A cold normally clears up in a week or so; flu symptoms are usually past their worst after 4–5 days, but you may feel tired and weak for up to several weeks afterward. There are ways to ease the symptoms:

- Keep warm and drink lots of liquids, especially water and fresh fruit juice.
- Take over-the-counter painkillers to help ease headaches and joint or muscle pain.
- 1,000 mg of Vitamin C 2 times a day taken at the onset of a cold may decrease the severity and duration of the cold.
- Over-the-counter cough medicines can help in the short term, but they only suppress the urge to cough—they don't cure it. Use them for nighttime relief only, and not longer than 7–10 days. Drinking a lot of water can help loosen phlegm as much as an expectorant cough syrup does.

Vaccinations against the flu are available, but are not 100 percent successful. They are generally administered once a year and are highly recommended for people over 65 years and people with certain chronic illnesses.

CALL A DOCTOR IF

- Your cough lasts more than a week
- A fever lasts longer than 3 days, or if symptoms include a severe headache, a stiff neck, abdominal pain, or pain urinating
- The person suffering from a high fever is a baby under 6 months old, an elderly person, or a child with a history of convulsions

Warning!

If a cough is accompanied by a high fever, difficulty in breathing, blue tongue or lips, drowsiness, or difficulty in speaking, call a doctor at once.

AROMATHERAPY

Steam inhalations of menthol, eucalyptus, or peppermint oil help clear a blocked nose. Pour a few drops into a bowl of very hot water, cover your head with a towel, and breathe in the vapor for 5 minutes or so.

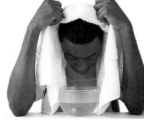

A steam inhalation can clear a blocked nose.

FEVERS

A fever is a temperature above 98.6°F (37°C). It is a common symptom of the flu and many other illnesses. It may be accompanied by shivering, sweating, headache, thirst, and flushed skin.

Many over-the-counter painkillers—such as aspirin—help relieve a fever. If you have a bacterial infection, your doctor may prescribe antibiotics. Drink plenty of fluids to replace those lost as sweat. Do not wear too many clothes, cover up with too many blankets, or have the room too hot.

Warning! Never give aspirin to a child under 12 years of age.

SORE THROATS

- Irritation, a tickling sensation, a feeling of heat or "rawness" at the back of the throat
- Visible redness at the back of the throat
- Tenderness in the neck

STREP THROAT:
- A fever above 101°F (39°C)

CALL A DOCTOR IF

- A sore throat lasts more than a few days
- You have a temperature over 101°F (39°C), but no other flulike symptoms
- You have trouble breathing or swallowing

The expression "sore throat" is self-explanatory, and almost everyone gets one from time to time. Usually sore throats are not much more than an irritation, but occasionally they can be serious and require medical treatment.

CAUSES
- Viral infections, such as colds, the flu, and chicken pox, can cause a sore throat.
- Bacterial infections, including whooping cough, can lead to a sore throat. One type of bacteria—beta-hemolytic streptococci—can cause "strep throat," a severe sore throat that, if left unchecked, occasionally has serious complications.

WHAT YOUR DOCTOR WOULD DO
Most sore throats clear up by themselves. To ease the soreness, you can gargle with an antiseptic solution, rest, and drink plenty of fluids (but avoid fizzy, carbonated drinks, which can irritate the throat). Using a humidifier in your bedroom will help to keep your throat moist.

If your doctor suspects that you have a bacterial infection, a swab may be taken from your throat and sent to a laboratory to be tested for bacteria. If necessary, your doctor will prescribe antibiotics.

ALTERNATIVE TREATMENTS

HOMEOPATHY
Throat pain soothed by warm drinks, especially if on the right side, may respond to 2 pellets of 12c *Lycopodium* every half hour up to 6 times as needed.

Lycopodium

HERBAL REMEDIES
- Garlic capsules or raw garlic both boost the immune system, keeping infection at bay. Alternatively, try sage, chamomile, or licorice tea to soothe a sore throat. **Warning!** Avoid sage tea if pregnant.

ACUPRESSURE
- Press your left thumb on the middle of the pad at the base of your right thumb for 1 minute and release. Repeat on the other hand.
- Using your thumb, press the sole of your foot in the depression under the ball of the foot for 1 minute.

Acupressure point on the sole of the foot, beneath the ball

TONSILLITIS & LARYNGITIS

CAUSES
■ A cold or flu virus or the same bacteria that can cause a "strep throat" can cause tonsillitis.
■ Laryngitis may be caused by a viral or bacterial infection, allergy, breathing in chemical vapor, or overusing your voice.

WHAT YOUR DOCTOR WOULD DO
In both cases your doctor may recommend bed rest with plenty of fluids, and over-the-counter painkillers if necessary. You may also be given antibiotics for a bacterial infection or antihistamines for an allergy.

SYMPTOMS

TONSILLITIS:
■ Sore throat
■ Hard to swallow
■ Fever
■ Spots on the tonsils or a white discharge
■ Headache

LARYNGITIS:
■ Hoarseness
■ Loss of voice
■ Sore throat
■ Fever
■ Cough

CALL A DOCTOR IF
■ A sore throat lasts more than a few days
■ Hoarseness lasts more than one week
■ You cough up phlegm

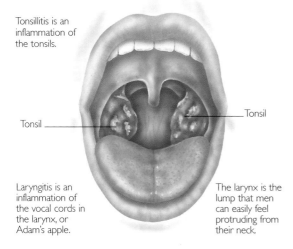

Tonsillitis is an inflammation of the tonsils.

Tonsil

Tonsil

Laryngitis is an inflammation of the vocal cords in the larynx, or Adam's apple.

The larynx is the lump that men can easily feel protruding from their neck.

ALTERNATIVE TREATMENTS

HERBAL REMEDIES
Elderflower taken as a tincture can help reduce inflammation. To prepare a tincture, half-fill a large screw-topped jar with the chopped herb, fill the jar with alcohol (vodka is ideal), and store away from direct sunlight. Shake the jar twice a day. After 2 weeks, strain the mixture into another jar. Store in a cool place. Take 10–30 drops straight or mixed with water, up to 4 times a day. **Warning!** Do not give tinctures to children.

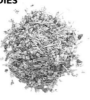

Elderflower

■ Or, gargle with warm tea made from red sage, bayberry, or white oak. Steep 1–2 teaspoons of the herb in a cup of hot water for 10 minutes and strain. Gargle with it several times a day. **Warning!** Do not use sage gargles in pregnancy.

HOMEOPATHY
■ *Spongia tosta* 2 pellets of 6 or 12c under the tongue every hour as needed up to 2 days is excellent for a barking cough.
■ *Rumex crispus* in the same dosage may be used if the cough is brought on by going from a warm room to the cold air or vice versa, with tickling in the throat.

ASTHMA

SYMPTOMS

- Wheezing
- A feeling of tightness in the chest
- Shortness of breath
- A cough, which may be dry or phlegmy
- Symptoms may be mild or severe

CAUSES

- One very common cause is an allergic reaction to one or more of several possible trigger substances, including animal hair, house dust, tobacco smoke, pollen, certain foods, and over-the-counter drugs like aspirin. Allergy-related asthma is often hereditary.
- Asthma may be brought on by emotional stress, exercise, and air pollution.
- Colds and lung infections can also cause asthma. ▶

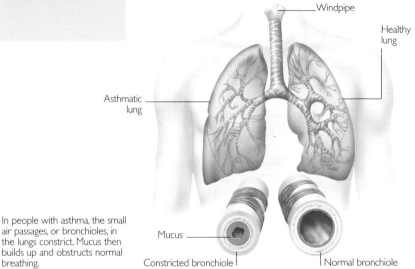

Windpipe

Healthy lung

Asthmatic lung

Mucus

In people with asthma, the small air passages, or bronchioles, in the lungs constrict. Mucus then builds up and obstructs normal breathing.

Constricted bronchiole

Normal bronchiole

ALTERNATIVE TREATMENTS

ACUPRESSURE

Try either of these pressure points if you think an asthma attack is about to start:
- Press your thumb at the acupressure point 2 fingers' width from the wrist

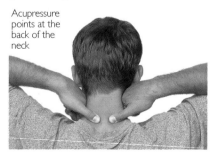

Acupressure points at the back of the neck

crease nearest the palm, on the inside of the forearm and in line with the thumb.
- Reach around behind your head and press each thumb gently on the acupressure points that are about a finger's width away from each side of the spine.

HOMEOPATHY

Asthma is a chronic illness best treated by Constitutional Homeopathy (see p.100) rather than symptomatic remedies:

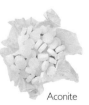

Aconite

WHAT YOUR DOCTOR WOULD DO

First your doctor will try to help you establish what triggers your asthma. If you don't know what brings it on, you may need to keep a diary so that you and your doctor can work out what is most likely to be the trigger. You will then be given advice on ways of eliminating the triggers or reducing their effects.

You may be prescribed a drug known as a bronchodilator, which helps open the narrowed airways in the lungs. This will either be taken by mouth, or from an inhaler. If your asthma is serious, your doctor may also prescribe a corticosteroid—a drug similar to a natural hormone in the body—which is useful both in preventing symptoms and as an emergency treatment for an attack.

If you smoke, your doctor will strongly recommend that you stop immediately. He may also give you advice on how to cope better with stress.

CALL A DOCTOR IF

- It is the first time you have had an attack
- Any drugs given do not work as soon as they should, or do not give you relief—new ones may be needed or the attack may be worse than usual

Warning!

Call for emergency help right away if an asthmatic complains of a suffocating feeling and finds it hard to talk; their nostrils flare; the skin between their ribs looks pulled in; and their nails or lips look bluish. This means they can't breathe in enough oxygen or breathe out enough carbon dioxide.

For a nighttime asthma attack accompanied by much anxiety, try *Arsenicum album* 30c potency 2 pellets under the tongue for 3–4 doses; or, take *Aconite* 6c as needed.

 ### HERBAL REMEDIES

An infusion of elecampane root may help a phlegmy chest. A mullein infusion may soothe a nighttime cough and help you sleep. To prepare an infusion, steep an herbal tea-bag or a teaspoon of the dried herb in a cup of boiling water for 5 minutes (then strain, if using dried herbs). You can add honey if you like.

REFLEXOLOGY

You may find some relief from asthma by applying pressure with your thumb on the lower part of the ball of the foot. You can find the point by following an imaginary line down from between the big toe and its neighboring toe (the toes here are spread apart for clarity).

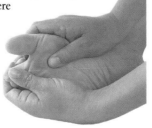

Reflexology point below the ball of the foot

BRONCHITIS

SYMPTOMS

ACUTE BRONCHITIS:
- A hacking cough
- White, yellow, or green phlegm
- Fever
- A sore, tight chest
- Pain when breathing deeply

CHRONIC BRONCHITIS:
- A cough that persists for 3 months at a time
- White, yellow, or green phlegm

CALL A DOCTOR IF

- A cough persists for more than a week
- You cough up white, yellow, or green phlegm
- You experience breathing difficulties

Bronchitis develops when the airways that connect the windpipe to the lungs become inflamed. There are two kinds: acute and chronic. Acute bronchitis shouldn't last for more than two weeks, but it can be dangerous in elderly people. Chronic bronchitis is more serious and may last for months.

CAUSES
- Viral infections are the most common cause of acute bronchitis, although bacteria are responsible in 10 percent of people.
- Cigarette smoking over time is the most common cause of chronic bronchitis.
- Repeated bouts of acute bronchitis can also lead to chronic bronchitis.
- Air pollution and exposure to certain industrial dusts or gases can increase coughing, mucus, and shortness of breath in people with chronic bronchitis.

WHAT YOUR DOCTOR WOULD DO
For acute bronchitis, the doctor may prescribe antibiotics or advise taking over-the-counter cough medicines, painkillers, resting, and drinking fluids.

For chronic bronchitis, a doctor may recommend yearly vaccinations to prevent the flu, and a once-only vaccination to prevent pneumonia, or you may be prescribed drugs to open up the airways. Anyone who suffers from bronchitis should stop smoking.

ALTERNATIVE TREATMENTS

HOMEOPATHY
- For a painful, hoarse voice, with coughing when talking, laughing, or breathing deeply, try *Phosphorus* 6 or 12c 2 pellets under the tongue every 4 hours up to 6 doses.
- If the cough is so painful you must hold your chest or your head with your hands, try *Bryonia alba* in the same dosage.

HERBAL REMEDIES
- Coltsfoot can relax tightened passages and mullein may have anti-inflammatory properties. To take either of these, make an infusion by steeping 1–2 teaspoons of the dried herb in a cup of boiling water for 10 minutes, then strain. Drink the infusion while it is still hot 3 times daily.
- To boost your immune system, take garlic daily, raw or in capsule form.

AROMATHERAPY
To improve breathing, try inhalations of steam scented with eucalyptus, lavender, rosemary, or hyssop. Pour a few drops of the essential oil into a bowl of boiling water. Inhale the vapor for 5 minutes. Or, put a few drops of oil onto a handkerchief and inhale. **Warning!** Do not use hyssop oil in pregnancy.

Digestive Problems

DIGESTIVE PROBLEMS

The food you eat is processed in your digestive system, starting in the mouth. As you chew, your teeth grind the food into smaller pieces and saliva begins to break it down. From the mouth, food travels through the gastrointestinal tract, which consists of the esophagus, stomach, and small and large intestines. In this tract food is further churned and processed with a variety of enzymes to extract the nutrients before the waste is expelled.

This complicated system does not always run smoothly, and there are many factors that can cause problems. An infection can cause nausea or diarrhea, and alcohol consumption and smoking can cause indigestion. Occasionally a food can cause an allergic reaction, and emotional stress can disrupt any and all aspects of digestive function, leading to pain, gas, bloating, or irregular bowel movements.

2

INDIGESTION & HEARTBURN

SYMPTOMS

INDIGESTION:
- Abdominal pain
- Belching
- Nausea
- Flatulence (gas)
- Vomiting

HEARTBURN:
- As for indigestion, but with the addition of a painful, burning sensation in the chest

CALL A DOCTOR IF

- Abdominal pain lasts more than 6 hours or is severe
- You vomit blood or pass a very dark stool
- You feel dizzy, faint, or feverish

Indigestion is a general term for various stomach problems brought on by eating; heartburn is a type of indigestion in which stomach acid enters the throat and causes irritation.

CAUSES
- Both complaints are often brought on by eating too much, too quickly, by eating rich or spicy foods, by drinking too much alcohol or coffee.
- Being seriously overweight may cause indigestion.
- Stress is also a cause of indigestion, as is smoking.
- Frequent indigestion may result from a bacterial infection associated with a peptic ulcer.
- Some pain-relievers can cause indigestion.
- A weak muscular valve around the stomach entrance can lead to heartburn.

WHAT YOUR DOCTOR WOULD DO
Some foods relax the stomach opening enough to promote heartburn in susceptible people, and your doctor will ask you to strictly avoid them for the healing period. If there is no serious cause for your indigestion or heartburn, your doctor may suggest antacid tablets. But if you are in danger of developing an ulcer from the excess stomach acid of indigestion, a medicine that protects the stomach from acid may be recommended. If a bacterial infection is to blame, antibiotics will be prescribed.

ALTERNATIVE TREATMENTS

HOMEOPATHY
- If the heartburn is eased by hot drinks, try *Arsenicum album* 6 or 12c 2 pellets up to 3 times every 15 minutes.

AROMATHERAPY
Massage is good for digestive problems because it can help the circulation in the stomach area. It also happens to be a good way to relax, which is also beneficial for people with indigestion. The essential oils of bergamot, chamomile, fennel, melissa, and peppermint are all good for aiding indigestion. Using light pressure, massage one of the recommended essential oils on the abdomen in a clockwise direction. **Warning!** Do not have a stomach massage if you have diverticultis, Crohn's disease, ulcers, cancer, or if you are pregnant.

Stomach massage stimulates circulation and can alleviate indigestion.

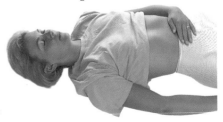

FLATULENCE (GAS)

SYMPTOMS

- A bloated feeling
- A frequent need to burp or pass gas
- Abdominal pain

CALL A DOCTOR IF

- Symptoms last more than 3 days: they could indicate an ulcer, hiatus hernia, irritable bowel, or lactose intolerance

Gas normally builds up in the body and needs to find a way out. This is normal and usually a minor problem, but in some cases it can possibly lead to extreme discomfort.

CAUSES

- Swallowing too much air when eating, drinking carbonated beverages, chewing gum, swallowing a lot when wearing false teeth, or feeling nervous can cause gas.
- Eating high-fiber foods, including beans, certain other vegetables and fruits, can cause gas.
- Gas can be a painful problem in people with lactose intolerance who do not have the enzyme needed to digest sugar (lactose) in dairy foods.
- Gas can also result from an infection in the digestive system.

WHAT YOUR DOCTOR WOULD DO

You can usually relieve gas without a doctor's help. Chewing food slowly, eating moderate amounts, sitting up straight when eating, and avoiding foods and beverages that cause the problem all help. Over-the-counter medicines can break up the gas from legumes such as baked beans. Tablets and drops of lactose—the enzyme needed to digest lactone—allow lactose-intolerant people to eat dairy products.

ALTERNATIVE TREATMENTS

ACUPRESSURE

With the thumb and index finger of one hand, squeeze the web of skin between the thumb and index finger of the other hand; repeat on the other hand. **Warning!** Do not do this if you are pregnant.

HERBAL REMEDIES

Chamomile and peppermint teas can soothe indigestion. Eating garlic, caraway seeds, and cloves, and using thyme and marjoram in cooking, can also help. Garlic is best raw, but is available in capsules.

HICCUPS

Hiccups are caused by spasms of the diaphragm, which lies beneath the rib cage. They may be caused by eating or drinking too much or too fast, or by drinking alcohol.

They usually go away on their own accord, but if they persist, try holding your breath, drinking water from the far rim of a glass, or breathing in and out of a paper bag (do not do this for more than 3 minutes). Or, try drinking a cup of lemon balm tea or peppermint tea.

Warning! See your doctor if hiccups last for more than a day.

NAUSEA & VOMITING

SYMPTOMS

- Nausea is a feeling of wanting to vomit but not necessarily actually doing so
- A wave of heat followed by a cold clamminess followed by vomiting

MOTION SICKNESS:
- Sweating and dizziness, along with nausea, when traveling

Nausea is one of the most common ailments and sometimes, but not always, leads to vomiting. Vomiting occurs when involuntary muscle spasms force the stomach to eject its contents through the mouth.

CAUSES

- Both nausea and vomiting can be caused by eating food that has begun to decay or to which you are allergic.
- People with the flu or other infections may experience nausea and vomiting.
- A disturbance in your balance can make you feel sick or vomit. This often occurs in the form of motion sickness; when you travel by car, bus, boat, or plane, what you see doesn't match up with what the balance mechanism in your ear senses and this has rapid consequences in some people.
- Nausea and vomiting is common in early pregnancy (see pp.80–81).
- Two of the symptoms of migraine headaches are nausea and vomiting.
- Certain serious complaints, such as hepatitis, uncontrolled diabetes, and appendicitis, can cause nausea and vomiting. ▶

ALTERNATIVE TREATMENTS

HERBAL REMEDIES

- Ginger root can be used to decrease the nausea of morning sickness, motion sickness, or an upset stomach. The adult dose of the powdered herb is 250 g (2 capsules) 3–4 times per day.

Ginger root is an old remedy for nausea.

HOMEOPATHY

- If you are retching and straining more than you are vomiting, try *Nux vomica* 6 or 12c 2 pellets up to every 5 minutes as needed, for no more than a few hours.

- If nausea and vomiting accompanies a cold with cough, try *Ipecac* 12 or 30c 2 pellets every 4 hours up to 4 doses as needed.

ACUPRESSURE

- For relief from nausea, firmly press your thumb 2 fingers' width below the crease on your wrist for 1 minute, 2 to 3 times. Repeat on the other wrist. Wrist bands are available that apply pressure to these points.

Point below the wrist

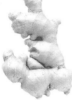

WHAT YOUR DOCTOR WOULD DO

Treatment for nausea depends on the cause. If it is due to a migraine or an infection, then your doctor will prescribe the appropriate treatments. If it is caused by food poisoning, she may recommend drinking plenty of water and avoiding eating anything but very plain food, such as dry toast or crackers, for a day or so until you feel better. Persistent vomiting or vomiting blood will require further investigation to establish the cause.

If you suffer from motion sickness, try sitting where the vehicle is steadiest—in the front seat of the car or bus, as close as possible to the wings of the plane or in the forward or middle cabin of a boat—and looking at the horizon or keeping your eyes closed. Always sit facing the direction of travel. Don't read or do anything that involves looking down for any length of time. Eat little and often before traveling, avoid fatty foods, and drink plenty of liquids, but not orange juice and coffee (which may irritate the stomach).

Your doctor may recommend an over-the-counter medicine to take before traveling or, for long trips, may suggest a skin patch that releases an anti-nausea medicine over a period of time.

CALL A DOCTOR IF

- Nausea and vomiting are accompanied by severe abdominal pain, a headache, blurred vision, a rash, or fever.
- Vomiting and diarrhea persist for more than 24 hours.
- You are taking a new medicine.

2

Warning!
Call the doctor if you vomit blood or a dark substance resembling coffee grounds or if your baby cannot keep any milk down.

- For motion sickness, help your balance mechanism by pressing your index finger in the hollow at the back of your jawline. Hold it lightly for 1 minute and breathe deeply. Repeat up to 2 times.

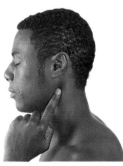

Point for motion sickness just below the ear

STOMACH ACHES

There are many causes of stomach ache, including eating spoiled food, viral infections, stress, or allergic reactions. Severe abdominal pain may have a more serious cause, such as a peptic ulcer or appendicitis.

Your doctor's treatment will depend on the cause. If it is not serious, you may be advised to change your diet or to learn to manage stress. Resting with a heating pad on the sore area may ease pain. Acute or persistent pain may require further investigation.

Warning! Call a doctor at once if you have severe prolonged stomach pain.

REACTIONS TO FOOD

2

SYMPTOMS

ALLERGY:
- Upset stomach with cramps
- Vomiting and/or diarrhea
- Breathing difficulties
- Swelling of the face, lips, tongue, and throat

INTOLERANCE:
- Uncomfortably full or bloated feeling
- Vomiting and/or diarrhea
- Gas
- Indigestion and/or heartburn

Many people believe they are allergic to certain foods when, in fact, they have an intolerance. The symptoms are sometimes similar. True food allergies are uncommon.

CAUSES
- A food allergy is a response of the body's immune system to one or more trigger foods—or allergens.
- If you have a food intolerance, you will feel unwell when you eat a certain food because your body lacks the enzymes that allow you to digest them.

WHAT YOUR DOCTOR WOULD DO
If you think certain foods may upset you, keep a diary of what you eat and how you feel. Your doctor can run tests to work out which foods don't agree with you. Ask other family members if anyone else has asthma, eczema, hay fever, or a food allergy because allergies tend to run in families.

Tablets and drops are available to help people with a milk sugar (lactose) intolerance to digest dairy products. Otherwise, the only treatment for food allergy or intolerance is to avoid eating the food that makes you unwell. If you are going to a restaurant, ask about ingredients before you order. Check ingredients on food labels when shopping.

ALTERNATIVE TREATMENTS

ACUPRESSURE
To help boost the immune system, place your thumb on the top of your left forearm, 2 thumbs' width from the wrist joint and press firmly. Repeat on the other arm.

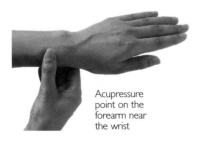

Acupressure point on the forearm near the wrist

ANAPHYLACTIC SHOCK

This is a very serious allergic reaction to a trigger substance such as peanuts, bee stings, shellfish, and certain drugs such as aspirin or penicillin. The symptoms include itching and swelling of the mouth, throat, and tongue, and a rash all over the body. The victim may become unconscious and could even die. Treatment is with an epinephrine injection, and many people with a serious allergy carry a pre-loaded syringe of epinephrine wherever they go. If you think someone is in anaphylactic shock, call 911 and give immediate first aid.

FOODS AND SYMPTOMS

FOOD TRIGGERS	SYMPTOMS
DAIRY PRODUCTS Milk, cheese, yogurt, cream, ice cream, cream soups, and certain baked goods and desserts.	**ALLERGY** Constipation, diarrhea, and vomiting; occasionally a rash and breathing problems. **INTOLERANCE** Bloating, cramps, and gas.
EGGS (ESPECIALLY THE WHITES) Eggs are in certain desserts—cakes, ice cream, mousses, and sherbets—mayonnaise, salad dressing, waffles, and pancakes.	**ALLERGY** A rash or intestinal upset. In some susceptible people, eggs cause asthma and eczema.
FISH Fresh, canned, smoked, or pickled fish, caviar, foods containing fish such as bisques, broths, and stews.	**ALLERGY** A rash, red itchy eyes, or a runny nose. Can cause asthma, diarrhea, and even anaphylaxis.
SHELLFISH Shrimp, mussels, crab, lobster, crayfish, clams, oysters, scallops, and seafood dishes.	**ALLERGY** A migraine, nausea, intestinal upset, rash, swelling of the skin, and anaphylaxis.
WHEAT Can be found in cereals, bread products, dry soup mixes and gravies, cakes, pasta, dumplings, and products containing flour.	**ALLERGY** Diarrhea and other intestinal upsets, migraine, and eczema. **INTOLERANCE** Bloating, cramps, diarrhea, pale foul-smelling bowel motions.
CORN Some soups and stews, baby foods (with cornstarch), baking mixes, processed meats, corn oils, margarine, salad dressings, and certain baked goods.	**ALLERGY** Rash, breathing problems, diarrhea, and other intestinal upsets; possibly anaphylaxis.
NUTS AND PEANUTS Candy and baked goods with pecans, walnuts, almonds, cashews, filberts, pistachios, and peanuts; oils from nuts.	**ALLERGY** Intestinal upsets and breathing problems; possible anaphylaxis.
FRUITS Citrus fruits, melons, and certain other fruits.	**ALLERGY** Rash on the face, itching or tingling in the mouth.
CHOCOLATE Confectionery, baked goods, and other products containing cocoa.	**ALLERGY** Rash.

CALL A DOCTOR IF

- You have violent stomach cramps, vomiting, diarrhea, or continued bloating

CALL 911 URGENTLY IF:
- Breathing becomes difficult or painful
- Your skin becomes flushed, itchy, and develops hives—this could be a sign of anaphylatic shock (see box on opposite page), which requires emergency medical treatment

2

Warning!
Use caution in trying an elimination diet on your own—it is easier and safer to ask for help from your doctor or a dietitian before you try cutting out any foods you think may be a problem.

DIARRHEA

- Frequent, watery, or loose bowel movements over which you have little control
- Abdominal cramps

2

Diarrhea is usually a minor complaint and almost everyone experiences it now and then. It normally clears up in a day or two by itself.

CAUSES

- Diarrhea is most frequently caused by viruses or food poisoning.
- Stress and anxiety may also be to blame.
- Drinking too much coffee can sometimes cause diarrhea.
- Diarrhea can be a reaction to some types of medicines; check with your doctor if it becomes severe or persistent.
- A food intolerance or allergy (see pp.30–31) can cause diarrhea.
- With viral diarrhea the symptoms will clear up in a few days.
- Food poisoning usually resolves in 24–48 hours.
- You may get diarrhea on vacation in another country for two reasons: either because you have eaten or drunk contaminated food or water, or simply because the harmless bacteria that normally live in your stomach are not the same as those that you ingest when you are in other countries. This can cause your stomach to be upset until it gets used to the new balance of bacteria. ▶

ALTERNATIVE TREATMENTS

HOMEOPATHY

For simultaneous vomiting and diarrhea, either *Arsenicum album* or *Veratrum album* in a 12 or 30c potency 2 pellets every half hour up to 4 doses.

HERBAL REMEDIES

- Infusions of agrimony, plantain, or geranium are suggested. To make an infusion, steep a teaspoon of the herb in a cup of hot water for 10 minutes, then strain. You can take 3–4 tablespoons 3 times daily.
- Peppermint or chamomile tea may be soothing as well.

The dried leaves of the peppermint plant are used to make a soothing tea.

VISUALIZATION

This can help you deal with the stress that may lead to diarrhea. Take the phone off the hook. Lie down or sit comfortably and close your eyes. Imagine yourself in a pleasant, peaceful place, such as on a beach, for 15 minutes. Or, close your eyes, breathe deeply, and listen to soothing music for half an hour.

WHAT YOUR DOCTOR WOULD DO

Except in severe cases, diarrhea does not need medical treatment. To avoid dehydration—when your body loses too much fluid—it is important to replace the fluids and salts in the body lost when you've got diarrhea. Children in particular are at risk of dehydration. You can buy suitable "oral rehydration" mixtures or you can make your own. Dissolve ½ teaspoon of salt and 8 teaspoons of sugar in 4 cups (1 liter) of clean water. Measure the amounts carefully. If you have a large enough container you can make larger quantities at a time, but be sure to keep the proportions accurate. Drink 1¾ cups (450 ml) every hour and eat no solid food until the diarrhea goes away.

Once you feel ready to eat solid foods, start off with bland ones. Doctors often recommend bananas, rice, and stewed apple. Drinking the water strained from boiled rice can be helpful, as can eating yogurt with live bacterial cultures.

Sensible precautions when traveling overseas include drinking only bottled water and avoiding ice cubes in your drinks. Avoid salads, wash and peel fruit carefully, and don't eat food that has been kept warm for long.

CALL A DOCTOR IF

- Abdominal pain or severe discomfort accompanies the diarrhea
- Diarrhea lasts longer than 48 hours (24 hours for children)
- The stool is black or bloody
- Diarrhea occurs with a fever of 101°F (39°C) or higher, chills, vomiting, or fainting

2

ACUPRESSURE

- Place your fingers on the inside of the leg, about 4 fingers' width above the inner ankle and just behind the shin bone. Massage in an upward movement.
  - Place one fingertip on your abdomen, about 3 fingers' width from your belly button, and massage gently in a circular motion.

Acupressure point above the ankle

REFLEXOLOGY

The areas said to help the digestive system are on the sole of the foot, just above the heel. Apply pressure to the reflexology point for the small intestine as shown; then work on either side of this point to soothe the large intestine.

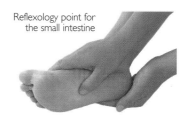

Reflexology point for the small intestine

CONSTIPATION

SYMPTOMS

- Bowel movements occur infrequently—as rarely as once every 3 days in adults, or every 4 days in children
- Bowel movements are difficult and painful
- Stool is hard and compact

Constipation means different things to different people simply because normal bowel movements vary from individual to individual. In general, a person is "regular," or has normal bowel movements, when a stool is passed anywhere between as often as three times a day to as little as once every three days. Constipation occurs when there is a change in the normal pattern and when the stool is so hard that it's uncomfortable to pass it.

CAUSES
- The main reason people suffer from constipation is that they don't have enough fiber in their diets. Fiber is found in foods such as fruit and vegetables, whole-wheat bread and pasta, and brown rice.
- Constipation can also be caused by a lack of water and other fluids in your diet.
- Not exercising enough can lead to constipation.
- People suffering from stress may sometimes develop constipation.
- Constipation can be caused by some vitamin supplements, such as iron and calcium, and by certain medicines, such as antihistamines.
- Pregnant women often become constipated.
- If constipation is persistent, it can be a symptom of a more serious disease. ▶

ALTERNATIVE TREATMENTS

HERBAL REMEDIES
- An infusion made from dandelion leaves acts as a gentle laxative. Steep 1–2 teaspoons of the dried leaves in a cup of hot water for 10 minutes, then strain. Stronger herbs, such as senna and cascara, can have side effects and should be used with professional supervision only.
- Trifala, (sometimes spelled triphala), made from the fruits of 3 different flowering herb trees, is a gentle, strengthening laxative considered to be an excellent health tonic in India. Take 2–3 tablets in the evening, with warm liquid. Trifala is safe for long-term use.

AROMATHERAPY
Mix 3 drops each of the essential oils of rosemary and marjoram and 2 drops of chamomile in 6 teaspoons (30 ml) of warmed almond carrier oil. Gently massage in a clockwise direction around the belly button, first applying light pressure and then releasing it.

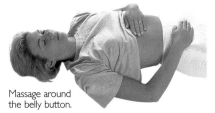

Massage around the belly button.

WHAT YOUR DOCTOR WOULD DO

Your doctor will ask some routine questions to rule out any serious cause for constipation—for example, you may be asked whether there is any blood in your stool. You will then be given advice about your diet and lifestyle. Fiber supplements are a safe way to prevent and treat constipation.

For more severe constipation, an occasional dose of milk of magnesia, mineral oil, glycerin, a glycerin suppository, or an enema is generally safe. If used too often, however, they can make the bowels "lazy" or hide a serious problem. It is much healthier to follow these self-help measures:

■ Eat at least five portions of fresh fruit, salad, and vegetables every day.

■ Switch to whole-wheat bread, and eat plenty of beans, brown rice, and whole-wheat pasta.

■ Minimize hard cheeses, white-flour breads and pastries, and meat. These three categories of foods are among the most constipating in the typical American diet.

■ Most of us don't drink nearly enough fluid. Try to drink at least eight glasses of water or other fluid a day.

■ Try to take some form of brisk exercise at least five times a week for half an hour.

CALL A DOCTOR IF

■ Constipation persists for longer than a week
■ There is blood in your stool, or you have severe, prolonged or repeated abdominal pain, or a fever
■ Constipation starts shortly after you have begun new medication

2

REFLEXOLOGY

To relieve constipation, work on the pressure point said to relate to the intestines. Gently apply pressure to the center of the foot, above the heel. Massage the area for 10 minutes.

Massage in a circular motion.

■ Bend your arm, placing your hand on the opposite shoulder. Press the thumb of your other hand deeply into the outer edge of the elbow crease in the bent arm for 1 minute. Repeat on the other arm.

ACUPRESSURE

■ Press a fingertip on the back of the forearm, about 4 fingers' width from the wrist.

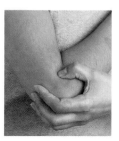

Acupressure point on the back of forearm

Acupressure point at the elbow

HEMORRHOIDS

2

SYMPTOMS

- Soreness and itching of the anal area
- A feeling of "fullness" around the anal area
- Bleeding from the anus
- Constipation
- A lump or swelling by the anus
- A discharge of mucus from the anus

Also known as piles, hemorrhoids are swollen veins that occur in the lining of the rectum and anus. Internal hemorrhoids develop in the rectum: normally, they can't be seen or felt, and the only symptom may be bleeding. Sometimes, however, they can prolapse, or fall down, into the anus, causing pain.

External hemorrhoids develop in the anus and are painful. These, too, may prolapse and protrude out of the anus. This type of prolapsed hemorrhoid can develop a blood clot, which may look serious and be painful, but should disappear on its own in about a week.

CAUSES

- Hemorrhoids often develop in people who are constipated (see pp.34–35) because straining to pass move the bowels puts pressure on the veins in the rectum and anus. Hard stools also irritate the veins.
- Pregnancy and childbirth can encourage hemorrhoids.
- People who stand or sit for long periods are more likely to develop hemorrhoids.
- Obesity can be a contributing factor. ▶

ALTERNATIVE TREATMENTS

HOMEOPATHY

Try one of the following Homeopathic remedies in a 30c potency 2 pellets under the tongue, repeated twice daily for up to 3 days.

- *Hamamelis* helps congested hemorrhoids oozing dark, thin blood for a long time.
- *Aesculus* helps if there are dry, sticking pains, worse when walking.

Hamamelis virginiana, witch hazel, the source for *Hamamelis*

HERBAL REMEDIES

- Try an ointment made from pilewort: simmer 2 tablespoons of the herb in 7 ounces (200 g) of petroleum jelly for 10 minutes. Cool before use.
- To reduce itching and pain, dab witch hazel on the area.
- You can use an infusion of yarrow (steep 1–2 teaspoons of the dried herb in a cup of hot water for 10 minutes) as a compress: dip a clean cloth or towel into the warm infusion and apply to the affected area until the cloth is cold.

Pilewort can be used in an ointment.

WHAT YOUR DOCTOR WOULD DO

The pain and swelling from mild hemorrhoids can be treated with over-the-counter ointments. Soft wiping cloths or a cool wet cloth can be used instead of toilet paper after bowel movements. Avoid straining. If your symptoms are more severe or if you have bleeding, see your doctor. Your doctor will need to examine the area, possibly by inserting a tube with a light on it, to rule out the possibility of more serious conditions.

Your doctor may prescribe a corticosteroid cream or suppositories to help reduce the swelling. Pills that soften the stool are sometimes given. Large and painful or prolapsed and bleeding hemorrhoids can be removed in the doctor's office using local anesthetics.

These are steps that you can take to help prevent hemorrhoids:
- Increase your intake of fiber: make sure you have five portions of fresh fruits and vegetables every day, and try to eat more legumes, whole-wheat bread, whole-wheat pasta, and brown rice.
- Try to drink at least eight glasses of water a day.
- Exercise at least twice a week for half an hour. This can help stop constipation, which can cause hemorrhoids.
- Try not to strain during bowel movements.

CALL A DOCTOR IF

- You have had anal bleeding and never had hemorrhoids before
- If you have chronic anal bleeding—either daily or weekly—even if you have already been diagnosed as having hemorrhoids

2

AROMATHERAPY

- Cypress, juniper, peppermint, and chamomile oils are recommended: mix a few drops of each of these essential oils into a carrier oil, such as almond or soybean, and apply to the affected area.
- Cypress, juniper, peppermint, and chamomile oils can also be used in a warm bath. Pour a few drops directly into the water.
- To relieve the constipation that can cause and irritate hemorrhoids, massage the stomach area with a mixture of 3 drops each of the essential oils of rosemary and marjoram and 2 drops of chamomile in 6 teaspoons (30 ml) of almond oil. Gently massage in a clockwise direction around the belly button, first applying pressure and then releasing it. **Warning!** Do not use juniper oil if pregnant.

Massage the abdomen in a clockwise direction.

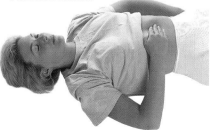

IRRITABLE BOWEL SYNDROME

2

SYMPTOMS

- Abdominal cramps
- Bloating
- Diarrhea or constipation
- Intestinal gas

Also known as spastic colon or irritable colon, irritable bowel syndrome (IBS) is a condition in which some of the muscles in the intestines and colon fail to move as they should—in synchronized contractions—and go into spasm instead. It is one of the most common digestive problems, affecting up to 20 percent of adults. It occurs more frequently in women than in men and usually starts in early adulthood.

The symptoms of IBS are sometimes—but not always—relieved by passing gas or having a bowel movement, but the sufferer may be left with the feeling that he or she has been unable to empty the bowels properly. It is common for symptoms to subside or disappear for some time, but attacks usually recur frequently.

CAUSES

No one knows for sure what causes IBS; the intestines are otherwise normal and there's no bleeding or unexplained weight loss.

- Stress is believed to be the main cause of IBS.
- An intolerance to certain foods may be another factor (see pp.30–31). ▶

ALTERNATIVE TREATMENTS

HOMEOPATHY

Irritable bowel syndrome is best treated by Constitutional prescribing, a remedy individualized to your total health picture, by a trained homeopath (see p.100). For relief of occasional urging that persists even after you move your bowels with cramping pain, try *Nux vomica* in a 30c potency 2 pellets repeated in 4 hours if necessary, up to 4 times.

HERBAL REMEDIES

Peppermint can help relax the intestines. You can make an infusion by steeping 1 teaspoon of the dried herb in a cup of boiling water for 30 minutes. Strain and drink 3 cups a day.

VISUALIZATION

To cope better under stress, close your eyes for 15 minutes and imagine yourself in a pleasant, peaceful place, such as on a

Lie down, relax your muscles, and visualize a quiet place.

WHAT YOUR DOCTOR WOULD DO

There is no test for irritable bowel syndrome, but your doctor will want to rule out other more serious conditions. You will be examined and the doctor may want to look inside your anus with a special light. Swabs may be taken, or you may be asked to bring in a stool sample.

There's no cure for irritable bowel syndrome, but your doctor can make suggestions on how you can try to reduce the symptoms:

■ After discussing your diet, the doctor may suggest you eat less fat and more fiber. Make sure you have five portions of fresh fruits and vegetables every day, and eat plenty of legumes, whole-wheat bread, and whole-wheat pasta, and brown rice.

■ Your doctor may ask you about your emotional state and how you deal with stress and may recommend several ways to reduce it.

■ In severe cases, your doctor may prescribe drugs that can reduce the spasms.

CALL A DOCTOR IF

■ You have abdominal pain accompanied by a fever of greater than 100.5°F (38°C)
■ There is blood in your stool
■ You have fevers and unexplained weight loss
■ There is a change in the frequency of your bowel movements
■ Mucus is present

2

---

deserted beach. Lying down helps, but you can also do this in a sitting position.

 REFLEXOLOGY

■ The reflexology point for your intestines is above the heel of the foot. To ease the symptoms of IBS, first apply pressure to the point, then massage the area for 10 minutes.
■ To reduce stress, massage the solar plexus point near the

Massaging this point reduces intestinal upsets.

Massage this point to reduce stress.

inside edge at the bottom of the ball of the big toe.

 ACUPRESSURE

To reduce pain, press your index fingers 2 fingers' widths' away from each side of your belly button for 1 minute and release; repeat 5 times.

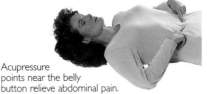

Acupressure points near the belly button relieve abdominal pain.

FOOD POISONING

SYMPTOMS

- Abdominal pain
- Vomiting
- Diarrhea

CALL A DOCTOR IF

- You have repeated bouts of vomiting
- Severe diarrhea lasts more than 48 hours for an adult, 24 for a child

Warning!
Call a doctor immediately if a person with food poisoning collapses.

This is a general name for any illness that results from eating spoiled food. The symptoms may be mild and last only a day or so, but in extreme cases they may be life-threatening.

CAUSES
- Eating food that has been contaminated with bacteria, viruses, or the poisons from them. Often everyone who ate the bad food becomes ill.
- One form of food poisoning is caused by *Salmonella* bacteria, which may be present in undercooked poultry, undercooked eggs, or foods made with raw eggs.

The *E. coli* bacteria, which are sometimes found in raw or undercooked meat can cause a severe form of food poisoning.

WHAT YOUR DOCTOR WOULD DO
Most food poisoning goes away after a few days and does not require medical treatment. You should avoid solid food for at least 24 hours and drink plenty of fluids.

If the vomiting and diarrhea are severe, the doctor may send samples to be analyzed. In the most severe cases, it may be necessary for the stomach to be cleaned out in the hospital, but most medical treatment concentrates on replacing lost fluids.

ALTERNATIVE TREATMENTS

 HERBAL REMEDIES
Ginger tea relieves nausea. Drink a cup every 2 hours; or take 2 ginger capsules.

HOMEOPATHY
- *Arsenicum album* 2 pellets of 12c potency every 15 minutes as needed, up to 12 times may help food poisoning with diarrhea and vomiting.

ACUPRESSURE
For nausea, apply pressure with your thumb on your inner forearm, 2 fingers' width below the wrist crease for 1 minute.

AVOIDING FOOD POISONING

- Always wash your hands with soap and water before handling food.
- Be careful when cutting meat: make sure you wash the surface where it was cut and the knife you used to cut it with, before bringing them into contact with other food. Wash your hands after touching raw meat. Don't let juices from raw meat drip onto other food in the refrigerator.
- Make sure frozen poultry is thawed completely and cooked right through.
- Never eat: mussels that do not open when boiled; food from cans that are bulging; food that smells or tastes bad.

Aches & Pains

ACHES & PAINS

At some point in your life, no matter how old you are, you will experience aches and pains, ranging from muscle cramps to back pain and gout. The musculoskeletal system consists of bones, muscles, ligaments, tendons, and joints, which can all cause pain if they are not working in harmony. Poor posture can put strain on the system, causing back pain, and repetitive movements such as working on a computer all day can result in pain in affected joints.

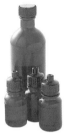

3

Some of these conditions, for example sprains, strains, and torn ligaments, may result from sudden exertion, not warming up before exercise, or from certain sports. Others affect the joints and include gout, rheumatoid arthritis, and osteoarthritis. Many aches and pains can be alleviated with rest, a change in diet, over-the-counter painkillers, or alternative therapies: some, however, may need surgery.

STRAINS & SPRAINS

SYMPTOMS

STRAINS:
- Pain
- Swelling
- Bruising

SPRAINS:
- Pain
- Some stiffness
- Immediate swelling

TORN KNEE OR ANKLE LIGAMENTS:
- Considerable pain
- The knee or ankle looks a strange shape
- You are unable to put any weight on the leg

TENDINITIS:
- Pain or tenderness
- Restricted movement of the muscle

CAUSES
- A strained muscle may result from sudden strenuous exertion or not warming up properly before exercise. Fibers are stretched or even torn, leading to bleeding in the damaged area.
- A sprain usually happens after a sudden, abnormal movement in that part of the body.
- Torn ligaments in the knee or ankle are a hazard of soccer and similar sports—a sudden twist of the joint while your weight is on that leg can do considerable damage.
- Tendinitis results from stressful movements repeated over and over at work or playing sports.

WHAT YOUR DOCTOR WOULD DO
For strains and sprains, doctors recommend RICE: rest, ice (applied to the area to reduce internal bleeding and swelling), compression (a carefully applied stretchy bandage), and elevation (raise it up to help prevent swelling). You may need anti-inflammatory painkillers.

Torn ligaments need surgical repair, or splinting to keep the joint immobile. Tendinitis generally responds to avoidance of the movement which caused it, or to improved positioning and frequent stretching during the movement as well as—in the short-term—anti-inflammatory drugs. ▶

ALTERNATIVE TREATMENTS

AROMATHERAPY
- For sprains, add 2 drops each of the essential oils of hyssop and sweet marjoram to a warm bath.
  - Or, massage the affected area with 2 drops each of

Apply a compress after massaging with oil.

hyssop and sweet marjoram oils mixed with a teaspoon of a carrier oil such as almond. Then apply a cold compress: add 5 drops of each of the essential oils to just enough water to soak a handkerchief or face cloth. You can cover the compress with plastic wrap to hold it in place. **Warning!** Do not use hyssop oil if pregnant.

HOMEOPATHY
- For muscle strains, take *Arnica* 30c every half hour, for 10 doses. Then take *Rhus toxicodendron* 6c 4 times a day until the pain disappears.

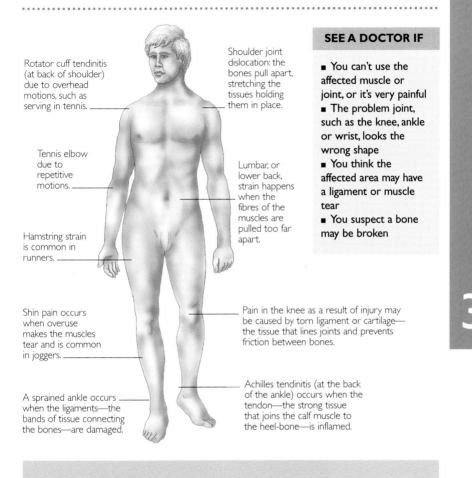

Rotator cuff tendinitis (at back of shoulder) due to overhead motions, such as serving in tennis.

Tennis elbow due to repetitive motions.

Hamstring strain is common in runners.

Shin pain occurs when overuse makes the muscles tear and is common in joggers.

A sprained ankle occurs when the ligaments—the bands of tissue connecting the bones—are damaged.

Shoulder joint dislocation: the bones pull apart, stretching the tissues holding them in place.

Lumbar, or lower back, strain happens when the fibres of the muscles are pulled too far apart.

Pain in the knee as a result of injury may be caused by torn ligament or cartilage—the tissue that lines joints and prevents friction between bones.

Achilles tendinitis (at the back of the ankle) occurs when the tendon—the strong tissue that joins the calf muscle to the heel-bone—is inflamed.

SEE A DOCTOR IF

- You can't use the affected muscle or joint, or it's very painful
- The problem joint, such as the knee, ankle or wrist, looks the wrong shape
- You think the affected area may have a ligament or muscle tear
- You suspect a bone may be broken

3

■ If you have a sprain or tendinitis, try *Arnica* 30c every half hour, for 10 doses, and follow with *Ruta* 6c 4 times a day until the pain subsides.

HERBAL REMEDIES
Comfrey helps to reduce swelling and bruising from sprains and strains. Make a compress by dipping a clean cloth in a cold comfrey infusion and applying to the affected area.

Use dried comfrey to reduce swelling.

(To make an infusion, steep 1–2 teaspoons of dried comfrey in a cup of hot water for about 10 minutes; then strain and cool.) Or, rub in some comfrey cream.

ACUPRESSURE
Apply gentle pressure approximately 6 inches (15 cm) away from the injury, not on the injury itself. For knee problems, find the pressure point on the outside of the leg, 4 fingers' width below the kneecap.

BURSITIS

SYMPTOMS

- Inflammation, swelling, and pain in a shoulder, elbow, hip, or knee following prolonged use of that joint
- Difficulty in moving the joint, with or without pain

CALL A DOCTOR IF

- Symptoms persist for more than a few days
- Anti-inflammatories or painkillers fail to reduce the swelling

CAUSES

- Bursitis is inflammation of the bursa, a fluid-filled pad that acts as a cushion where tendons or muscles cross bones. It happens when repeated pressure is put on a joint such as a knee, elbow, shoulder, or hip. It often occurs in people who participate in sports or manual labor.

WHAT YOUR DOCTOR WOULD DO

Rest the area as much as you can; the inflammation should go away by itself within about 10 days. Applying ice cold compresses to the area and taking over-the-counter anti-inflammatory painkillers will help with swelling and pain. In severe cases the doctor may need to inject anti-inflammatory drugs. Physical therapy can also help.

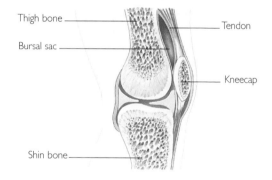

Thigh bone — Tendon

Bursal sac — Kneecap

Shin bone —

ALTERNATIVE TREATMENTS

HERBAL REMEDIES

To ease pain, rub a tincture of lobelia and cramp bark on the affected area. To make a tincture, half-fill a screw-top jar with the chopped or ground herbs, fill the jar with alcohol (vodka is ideal), and store in a warm dark place. Shake it twice a day. After 2 weeks, strain into another jar and store in a cool place.
- Bromelain, from pineapples, is an excellent anti-inflammatory medicine. Take 2 capsules on an empty stomach (if consumed with food, the bromelain will get "used up" in the stomach) 2 or 3 times daily for up to 5 days to relieve pain and swelling.

PREVENTING BURSITIS

- Always remember to warm up and cool down properly before and after doing any form of exercise. This will help to avoid putting unnecessary strain on your joints.
- When doing activities that require being on your knees, such as gardening, wear kneepads or use a foam rubber mat to help lessen the pressure on the kneecaps.
- If you have a problem with a particular joint, wear an elastic bandage to support it.

REPETITIVE STRAIN INJURY

SYMPTOMS

■ Pain, weakness, swelling, and burning in the affected area

CALL A DOCTOR IF

■ Pain is accompanied by stiffness in the hands or fingers and/or swollen joints
■ Pain in your wrist or hand occurs after a fall or other accident
■ Pain becomes worse at night
■ Your fingers and hands turn white and then red in cold weather

Also known as RSI, repetitive strain injury is a disorder that usually affects the hand, thumb, neck, elbow, and shoulder. Usually the sheath that surrounds a tendon (which attaches a muscle to a bone) becomes inflamed.

CAUSES

■ It is caused by overuse of the affected area and by poor posture. It is common in people who spend many hours at a computer keyboard, play a lot of sports, or do any repetitive physical work.

WHAT YOUR DOCTOR WOULD DO

Short-term treatments for RSI include rest, cold compresses, and anti-inflammatory painkillers. For example, for RSI of the hand and wrist, you may need to wear a splint and change your working practices. Make sure your chair is comfortable and pay attention to your posture. If you work at a computer, take a 10-minute break from the screen every hour. Your elbows should not rest below your wrists when your hands are on the keyboard. In the most severe cases of RSI, sufferers have found themselves unable to continue in their occupation, so take advice about preventive measures as soon as you notice any problem.

3

ALTERNATIVE TREATMENTS

HERBAL REMEDIES

Try a hot poultice made from comfrey, slippery elm, linseed, or marsh mallow:
■ Boil the fresh leaves of your chosen herb and when cool enough to handle, squeeze out any extra liquid. Apply the herbs directly to the affected area using a piece of gauze to keep the leaves in place.

Comfrey

Slippery elm

Marsh mallow

Linseed

■ You can use the dried herb by adding hot water to make a paste and holding it in place with gauze.

HOMEOPATHY

■ To relieve pain, rub *Arnica* cream into the affected area.
■ Take *Ruta* 12c or 30c 2 pellets under the tongue twice daily for 3–5 days.

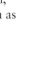

Rub *Arnica* cream onto unbroken skin only.

MUSCLE CRAMPS

SYMPTOMS

- Sudden stabbing pain which usually passes after a short while

RESTLESS LEGS

This is the name given to an uncomfortable syndrome in which the legs ache, feel hot, and uncomfortable and need to keep moving around. It often occurs at night, can run in families, and may be linked to smoking and caffeine consumption.

If it is severe, your doctor may prescribe drugs. Otherwise, if you smoke or drink a lot of coffee or cola, cut down or stop.

Cramps occur when muscles contract very tightly and don't release again as they should do—sometimes because the various chemicals in the muscles are out of balance. The muscle goes into a painful spasm and feels solid to the touch.

CAUSES

- Cramps often occur during or after exercise, which can cause a build-up of certain chemicals in the body.
- Excessive sweating can lead to cramps because of a chemical imbalance.
- Cramps can occur in the middle of the night. No one really knows what causes this, although poor circulation may be one explanation (this is different from restless legs; see box, left).

WHAT YOUR DOCTOR WOULD DO

There isn't a cure for cramps. The best treatment is to massage the area that hurts, warm it, and stretch it gently. To help prevent cramps, make sure you drink plenty of fluid (at least eight glasses a day), particularly in hot weather. To prevent getting cramps at night, try doing stretching exercises after having a warm bath before going to bed.

ALTERNATIVE TREATMENTS

 HERBAL REMEDIES
Ginkgo biloba can help ease cramps. Take a 60-mg capsule twice daily. **Warning!** Don't take ginkgo if you are on blood-thinners or take aspirin regularly.

ACUPRESSURE
For cramps in the calf, press firmly on the area at the lower end of the calf muscle for 2–3 minutes.

 AROMATHERAPY
Massage the affected muscle with a few drops each of the essential oils of

basil and marjoram, diluted in 2½ teaspoons of warmed almond oil.
Warning! Do not use these particular essential oils if pregnant.

HOMEOPATHY
For leg and foot cramps, at night, in bed, try *Causticum* 12c 2 pellets every 30 minutes up to 4 times.

Massage may help a muscle cramp.

3

NECK & SHOULDER PAIN

- A dull pain and difficulty in moving your head or shoulder

WHIPLASH:
- Sudden pain in the neck following an injury

CALL A DOCTOR IF

- Neck pain occurs after an accident
- Neck pain persists for longer than 1 day
- A stiff neck is accompanied by fever, severe headache, and vomiting—these could be symptoms of meningitis

Neck and shoulder pain are very common. Poor posture, muscle tension, and injuries strain the soft tissue, muscles, and joints of our necks and shoulders.

CAUSES
- Sleeping awkwardly, injury, and muscle tension from stress can cause pain and stiffness in the area.
- A sudden jerking of the neck can cause whiplash; this occurs most often in a car accident.
- Prolonged work on a computer, or improper keyboard height, monitor height, or other workstation factors, or cradling the telephone receiver between ear and neck, can all contribute to neck stiffness and pain.

WHAT YOUR DOCTOR WOULD DO
For stiffness and pain in the neck and shoulder, use hot or cold compresses or packs and take over-the-counter anti-inflammatory painkillers. If it is no better within 24 hours, see your doctor, who may recommend certain exercises. The doctor may need to rule out a more serious condition.

If you are in an accident and experience a neck injury, it is best to not move and call 911.

3

ALTERNATIVE TREATMENTS

ACUPRESSURE
- For neck pain, apply pressure with the tips of your index fingers pressing upward toward your head. There are 2 points between the bottom of

Acupressure points for neck pain (left) and shoulder pain (right)

the skull and the top of the neck muscles, each 2 fingers' width from the center of the vertebrae running down your neck.
- To relieve shoulder pain, press the point on the muscle midway between the point of your shoulder and your neck for up to 3 minutes.

AROMATHERAPY
Add a few drops of the essential oil of rosemary to bath water. Or mix the drops in 2½ teaspoons of a carrier oil, such as almond or soybean; massage it into the painful area.

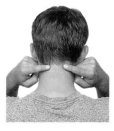
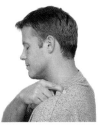

BACK PAIN

SYMPTOMS

LOW BACK PAIN:
- Pain in the lower back after strenuous activity or heavy lifting
- An ache in the lower or middle back after sitting or standing for long periods

BACK STRAIN:
- Pain and tenderness in larger back muscles

SCIATICA:
- Pain in the buttock and down the thigh, sometimes as far as the foot

DISK PAIN:
- Lower back pain, sometimes with sciatica
- Numbness and tingling

CAUSES
- **Low back pain** is usually caused by poor posture and sitting incorrectly; overexertion, improper lifting; the weight and the ligament relaxation of pregnancy; lack of sleep; stress.
- **Back strain** is the name sometimes given to muscle pain and stiffness and is often caused by tension and poor posture.
- **Sciatica** results from pressure on the sciatic nerve, usually from a tense muscle or a slipped disk.
- **Disk pain** may result from a slipped disk after sudden strenuous and awkward activity, but is more usually caused by wear and tear to the disks.

WHAT YOUR DOCTOR WOULD DO
Your doctor will examine you, rule out a urine infection, and, if necessary, arrange an X ray or scan.

For most back pain, the doctor will recommend anti-inflammatory painkillers, heat, and, perhaps, massage, careful stretching exercises, and other physical therapy. Rest is no longer recommended for most back pain. However, for a slipped disk some physicians advise several weeks of bed rest. ▶

ALTERNATIVE TREATMENTS

HOMEOPATHY
Take any of these in a 6 or 12c potency 2 pellets every 4 hours up to 5 days.
- *Hypericum perforatum* is helpful for injuries to the tip of the tailbone.
- *Arnica montana* is good for any bruise or blunt injury that is tender to the touch.
- *Bryonia alba* may help sharp shooting pain, worse from the slightest motion.
- If lying on a hard surface feels better, consider *Natrum muriaticum*.

ACUPRESSURE
- For low back pain, follow a line from the point between your little and ring fingers to just below your wrist and apply pressure for 3 minutes.
- Also for low back pain, press with both thumbs on either side of the spine just above the pelvis for 1 minute, then gently massage.

Acupressure point for low back pain

HERBAL REMEDIES
To make an infusion for one of the following teas, steep a tea bag or a teaspoon of the dried herb in a cup of

A slipped disk, or disk prolapse, occurs when the disk in the spine is injured. It is most common among people in their 30s. Most slipped disks occur in the lower back.

A kidney infection can cause pain in the area where the lowest ribs meet the spine. **Warning!** If you have pain here, call your doctor right away.

Back strain in the larger back muscles results from tension in the muscles.

Osteoarthritis may cause pain anywhere along the spine (see pp.50–51).

CALL A DOCTOR IF

- Back pain is accompanied by a fever of more than 100°F (38°C)
- There is tenderness of one of the bony prominences of the spine
- You have loss of bowel or bladder control
- You feel numbness or weakness in one or both arms or legs

Low back pain from lifting or over-activity typically involves either the middle of the lower curve, at the waistline, or else the area across the top of the pelvis, at the belt line.

Sciatica occurs when pressure on the nerve that runs from the base of the spine to the foot causes pain.

A fall can make the base of the spine, called the coccyx, painful.

3

---

boiling water for 5 minutes. Strain if necessary and add honey if you like.
- Try white willow for reducing pain.
- For sciatica, try white willow, black cohosh, skullcap, or rosemary.

AROMATHERAPY
A few drops of the essential oils of rosemary, chamomile, or lavender can be added to bath water. Or, mix the drops in 2½ teaspoons of a carrier oil, such as almond or soybean, and massage it into the affected area. In addition, try geranium oil for sciatica.

REFLEXOLOGY
For 1 minute, gently apply pressure to one of the reflexology points.

The point for the lower spine is on the inside edge of the foot.

The point for the middle spine area is by the ball of the foot, just below the big toe.

The upper spine point is near the big toe.

The point for sciatica runs across the heel.

OSTEOARTHRITIS

SYMPTOMS

- Pain and stiffness in a joint or joints with or without obvious swelling, particularly in the hip, knees, spine, and hands
- Eventually, difficulty in moving the joints
- In a few cases, muscle inflammation
- Rarely, extreme pain from muscle or nerve damage caused by bone spurs
- Absence of fever or heat in affected joints

CAUSES

- Doctors don't know exactly what causes osteoarthritis, although it affects more women than men and sometimes runs in some families. It can follow an injury to a joint. It is also generally thought to be part of getting older.
- If osteoarthritis causes joints to become deformed, they can develop an extra bony growth, known as spurs, which can press on surrounding muscles and nerves. ▶

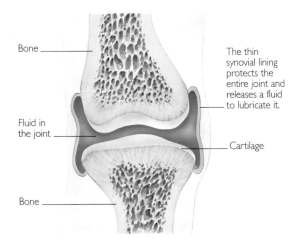

Bone

The thin synovial lining protects the entire joint and releases a fluid to lubricate it.

In a healthy joint, cartilage—a tough smooth tissue—covers the ends of bones where two of them meet, acting as a cushion.

Fluid in the joint

Cartilage

Bone

ALTERNATIVE TREATMENTS

HOMEOPATHY

Take 6c of one of these remedies 4 times daily, for up to 2 weeks.
- *Rhus toxicodendron* is recommended for pain with stiffness brought on by dampness and rest.
- *Bryonia* is suggested for severe pain with movement.

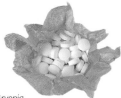

Bryonia

HERBAL REMEDIES

There are a few remedies that an herbalist may suggest to help relieve the symptoms of osteoarthritis. To make a tincture, half-fill a large screw-top jar with the herb, fill the jar with alcohol (vodka is ideal), and store in a warm place away from the sun. Shake the jar twice a day. After 2 weeks, strain the mixture into another jar and store in a cool place. ▶

Devil's claw can be used to make a tincture.

WHAT YOUR DOCTOR WOULD DO

Your doctor may take X rays to examine the bones for osteoarthritis. There is no cure, but treatments are aimed at reducing the pain. They include anti-inflammatory painkillers and perhaps injections into the affected joints. Applying heat to may be recommended. Glucosamine supplements can be used to relieve the pain of osteoarthritis. Gentle, regular exercise is a good idea because it keeps the muscles on either side of the affected joint in good condition. Physical therapy may also be suggested.

CALL A DOCTOR IF

- You develop severe pain or prolonged stiffness in your joints
- If your pain interferes with your daily activities

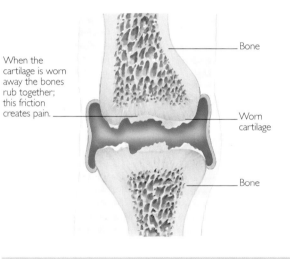

When the cartilage is worn away the bones rub together; this friction creates pain.

Bone

Worn cartilage

Bone

In osteoarthritis, the most common type of arthritis, the cartilage in the joint wears away after years of use. This is sometimes referred to as wear-and-tear arthritis.

3

- Take 1 tablespoon of a tincture made from devil's claw daily.
- For pain relief, try 1 teaspoon 3 times daily of a tincture of 2 parts willow and 1 part of nettle.
- To ease muscle tension, you can rub the affected area with a tincture of lobelia and cramp bark.

AROMATHERAPY

Gently massage the affected area with a few drops of tiger balm, chamomile, or lavender essential oil in 2½ teaspoons of a carrier oil such as almond or soybean.

REFLEXOLOGY

To relieve pain in the hip or knee joint, gently apply pressure for 1 minute to the relevant reflexology point shown below. Use the right foot for joints on the right side of the body, the left foot for those on the left side. **Warning!** Do not do this if you are pregnant.

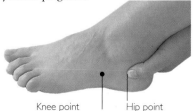

Knee point   Hip point

RHEUMATOID ARTHRITIS

SYMPTOMS

- Pain, swelling, warmth, and stiffness in the arms, legs, wrists, or fingers on both sides of the body
- Fatigue
- Symptoms are more severe on awakening
- In children, loss of appetite, fever, rash on the arms and legs

CALL A DOCTOR IF

- Joints suddenly become swollen, stiff, and painful
- A child has achy joints and a rash in the armpits, or on the wrists, knees, or ankles along with a fever

3

CAUSES

This condition is more common in women and often begins after 40 years of age, but can happen at any time. It is thought to be caused by a virus or other trigger causing the immune system to attack the body's own tissues.

WHAT YOUR DOCTOR WOULD DO

Your doctor may prescribe anti-inflammatory drugs and advise rest, heat compresses, and gentle exercise. Physical therapy can help relieve pain and give greater mobility. In extreme cases, surgery may be necessary to replace joints with artificial ones.

In rheumatoid arthritis, the synovial lining becomes inflamed and causes the cartilage to break down. (See p.50 for a healthy joint.)

The synovial lining thickens and becomes inflamed.

The joint looks swollen and misshapen.

The cartilage wears away.

Extra fluid puts pressure on the cartilage.

ALTERNATIVE TREATMENTS

HERBAL REMEDIES

To relieve the pain, try a tincture of willow bark. To prepare a tincture, half-fill a large screw-top jar with the herb, fill the jar up with alcohol (vodka is ideal), and store in a warm dark place. Shake the jar twice a day. After 2 weeks, strain into another jar and store in a cool place. Take 1 teaspoon 3 times daily.

HOMEOPATHY

Rheumatoid arthritis is a chronic, progressive illness. See a professional for a Constitutional prescription (see p.100).

AROMATHERAPY

Gently massage the joints with tiger balm, or use a few drops of chamomile or lavender essential oil diluted in a carrier oil such as almond or soybean.

Massage the oils into the affected joint.

GOUT

- Sudden, unexpected sharp pain in the joint of a big toe, ankle, finger, or knee that lasts no more than a week and may recur
- Swelling and inflammation in the affected joint, as well as a sensation of heat
- In an extreme case, fever and chills

CALL A DOCTOR IF

- Severe pain lasts more than 3 days or recurs, or if it occurs with fever and chills
- The symptoms increase while taking medicine that was prescribed for it by your doctor

Gout is a form of arthritis that mainly affects such joints as the big toe, knees, fingers, and elbows. It occurs when an extremely high level of uric acid in the blood creates crystals that become deposited in a joint. Gout is most common in middle-aged men.

CAUSES
- Men who are overweight or taking diuretics for high blood pressure are prone to gout.
- Heredity is a factor in half of the cases.
- An injury, surgery, stress, and reactions to alcohol and certain drugs, such as aspirin and antibiotics, can cause gout.
- Kidney disorders and enzyme deficiencies can lead to gout.
- Certain foods can trigger gout.

WHAT YOUR DOCTOR WOULD DO
Your doctor will probably suggest taking anti-inflammatory painkiller drugs. Drugs may also be given to help prevent the build-up of crystals, but it is possible to control this by what you eat. If you have gout, avoid eating organ meats, shellfish, processed meat, and fish (especially sardines), canned fish, asparagus, spinach, most types of dried beans, chocolate, beer, and red wine.

3

ALTERNATIVE TREATMENTS

 HOMEOPATHY
Ledum palustre may be helpful for a swollen big toe that is not red that feels better with cold application.
- Try *Bryonia alba* for gout that is worse from the slightest movement.

Homeopathic *Bryonia* is an effective painkiller.

Warning! If you are taking the medicine colchicine, do not try herbal remedies.

ACUPRESSURE
- Using your thumb, apply steady pressure just below the ball of the foot on the inside edge. Repeat on the other foot.
- Use your index fingers to apply pressure on each foot to the top of the webbing between the big and second toe.

HERBAL REMEDIES
To reduce uric acid, drink an infusion of gravelroot or celery seed 3 times daily. Steep 2 teaspoons of the herb in a cup of boiling water for 10 minutes.

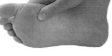
Acupressure point below ball of foot

CHRONIC PAIN

SYMPTOMS

- Persistent muscle pain, along with swelling, stiffness, and cramps
- Dull aching or sharp back pain, which is intermittent or continuous and localized or radiating
- Continuous joint pain and tenderness with restricted movement

OTHER RELATED SYMPTOMS:

- Muscle weakness
- Numbness, "pins and needles," or tenderness
- Difficulty sleeping
- Lack of energy
- Depression

The broad medical term "chronic pain" covers any pain that lasts for more than 6 months, despite medical treatment. The pain can be mild or excruciating. Sometimes it can be difficult to diagnose the cause.

CAUSES

- Any of a number of conditions related to the aging process, particularly ones that affect bones and joints, such as osteoarthritis, can cause chronic pain.
- Chronic pain can occur because of damage to the nerves from injuries or diseases that fail to heal.
- Chronic pain can be caused by poor posture or repeated movements.
- Having an injury such as a sprained ankle, or wearing high heels can cause joint or muscle pain elsewhere in the body. Lifting objects in the wrong way or lifting heavy objects can strain the back and cause back pain. Being overweight can put strain on the back and the knees.
- Certain diseases cause chronic pain, including cancer, multiple sclerosis, and peptic ulcers.
- Stress or other emotional problems can decrease the quantity of natural painkillers the body makes, increasing the level of pain felt. ▶

ALTERNATIVE TREATMENTS

AROMATHERAPY

Mix together a few drops of the following essential oils with 2½ teaspoons of a carrier oil, such as sweet almond, apricot kernel or jojoba oil. Massage at the site of your pain, rubbing the oil well into the skin.

- To reduce inflammation and relax muscles, use lavender oil.
- To bring down swelling and speed up healing, try eucalyptus oil.

For a massage, mix essential oils with a carrier oil

- To relieve the pain and stiffness of joint problems, try ginger oil.

ACUPRESSURE

Depending on where the pain is, a number of acupressure points can help reduce pain. Using the tip of your thumb or finger, apply pressure to the point for 1 minute.

Acupressure point above ankle for abdominal pain

WHAT YOUR DOCTOR WOULD DO

Your doctor will try to determine the cause of pain and treat you accordingly. For mild chronic pain, over-the-counter painkillers, such as aspirin may be recommended (though aspirin is unsafe for children). Stronger painkillers may be prescribed for more serious problems, and injections of a steroid drug may be recommended for some conditions.

Your doctor may recommend going to a pain clinic where specialists will help you learn how to control the pain; for example, through meditation and biofeedback techniques. In severe cases, TENS, or transcutaneous electrical nerve stimulation may be suggested. This is a small device with probes attached to the site of the pain to block any pain signals. You can apply the treatment yourself in the comfort of your own home. Some doctors prescribe low doses of antidepressants. These may block the chemical substances that are responsible for pain.

Hydrotherapy (water therapy) can be effective in the treatment of pain. One type, for example, involves applying alternate hot and cold compresses to the affected area. Another involves swimming or other gentle exercise in a warm hydrotherapy pool.

SEE A DOCTOR IF

- You have pain for several weeks and it continues after taking over-the-counter painkillers
- Pain doesn't respond to medicine prescribed by your doctor
- The symptoms of your chronic pain suddenly change

3

- For abdominal pain, place your thumb on the inside of your leg, 4 fingers' width above the ankle. Repeat on the other leg. **Warning!** Do not use this point if you are pregnant.
- To ease pain in the upper body, place your thumb on the top of your forearm, 2 fingers' width above the wrist. Repeat on the other arm; repeat the cycle 3 times.

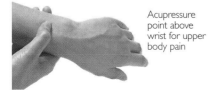

Acupressure point above wrist for upper body pain

HOMEOPATHY

Many different chronic physical and emotional problems can cause the body to experience pain. A consultation with a professional is advised. However;

- *Arnica* cream can reduce muscle and other pains not related to your joints.

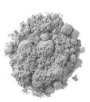

Potassium dichromate, the source of *Kali bichromicum*

- *Kali bichromicum* can reduce persistent pain and *Rhus toxicodendron* is good for back pain and pain related to joint problems including arthritis.

CHRONIC FATIGUE SYNDROME

SYMPTOMS

- Fatigue, muscle pain, and weakness
- Headaches
- Inability to concentrate
- Low fever
- Recurring sore throat
- Poor sleep

CALL A DOCTOR IF

- You are extremely fatigued with no clear reason

Warning!
Consult a specialist before taking herbal remedies—some of them can have adverse side effects.

Chronic fatigue syndrome (CFS) has many symptoms and can be difficult to diagnose, some doctors do not accept that CFS exists as a separate medical condition. It occurs most often in women under 45 although anyone can get it. The illness comes on suddenly and may last several years.

CAUSES
- No one knows what causes CFS, but research has shown that some sufferers have disturbances in their immune systems. One unproven theory is that a virus attacks the body when the person is already fatigued or stressed. Other theories include antibiotics and body changes from exposure to pesticides or other harmful chemicals, or a food allergy.

WHAT YOUR DOCTOR WOULD DO
There are no drugs specifically for the illness so your doctor will suggest ways of easing the symptoms, such as resting when necessary, getting exercise and making sure you have a healthy diet. Over-the-counter painkillers may help with aches and fevers in the short term. Some doctors prescribe antidepressants because, although there is no proof that CFS has a psychological basis, people with it may understandably become depressed.

ALTERNATIVE TREATMENTS

HOMEOPATHY
Treatments depend on the individual, so a consultation with a professional is advised.

AROMATHERAPY
Try lavender oil to reduce tiredness, weakness, and pain. Put a few drops on a tissue and inhale. Or, put 6 or 8 drops in a warm bath before you get in.

ACUPRESSURE

To reduce depression and fatigue and boost your immune system, try one of these pressure points.
- Using the tips of your middle fingers, gently apply pressure on the back of your neck at the hollows at the base of the skull, about 2 inches (5 cm) to each side of the spinal cord.
- Using the tip of your right middle finger, apply pressure about 2 inches (5 cm) from the base of your neck on your left shoulder; repeat on the other side. If you are pregnant, apply only light pressure.

SKIN & HAIR PROBLEMS

The largest organ of the human body is the skin. It protects the internal organs from outside invaders, such as germs and bacteria, and helps regulate body temperature through the sweat glands. Skin consists of several layers, one of which is keratin—the same material found in hair.

The outer layer of the skin is constantly being replaced in an almost unnoticeable way, but sometimes too many skin cells are produced, resulting in psoriasis; large flakes of dead skin on the scalp are known as dandruff. Some skin problems, such as eczema, are triggered by contact with an allergen, such as detergents. Although skin ailments are rarely life-threatening, they can sometimes cause discomfort, for example blisters and, because a healthy complexion is considered attractive, some, such as acne, can be embarrasing.

4

CUTS & BRUISES

SYMPTOMS

INFECTION:
- Redness, swelling, and pain
- A colored discharge
- Fever
- Swollen lymph nodes
- Red streaks spreading from the injury toward the heart

BRUISING:
- Discoloration of the skin: red, purple, or yellowish green

CALL A DOCTOR IF

- The wound is large or deep
- Underlying tissue, fat, or muscle is exposed
- Bleeding won't stop
- There are signs of infection, such as redness, pain, or pus

The skin protects us from infection, but can easily be cut or scraped. Bruising happens when there is bleeding under the skin.

CAUSES

- A cut, or incision, has a clean edge, usually from a knife or similar object. If the wound has jagged edges, it is called a laceration and the tissue is more damaged. If the skin is rubbed against a hard surface and is scraped away, the injury is called an abrasion.
- A bruise occurs when a part of the body suffers a sudden hard impact. It is normally minor, but very severe bruising can be life-threatening. Sometimes a bruise results from internal bleeding.

WHAT YOUR DOCTOR WOULD DO

Most wounds can be looked after safely at home. Stop the bleeding before you do anything else. Gently press with a sterile dressing until the bleeding stops. Large or deep cuts may need stitching by a doctor. Wash your hands, then clean the cut gently under warm running water, using a mild soap. Use an antiseptic wipe on the area, if there's a particular danger of infection, then dry the cut with a clean cloth or tissue and apply a clean bandage.

To treat a bruise, place an ice-pack, bag of frozen peas or a cold cloth on the area. Press lightly for up to 10 minutes to help reduce the pain and swelling.

4

ALTERNATIVE TREATMENTS

HOMEOPATHY
- For bruising, use *Arnica montana*. Try 2 pellets of 12c or 30c potency every 2 hours up to 24 as needed. Or gently rub the oil or cream into unbroken skin.
- For injuries to the fingertips or

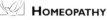
St John's wort is used to make *Hypericum*.

other nerve-rich areas, where pains shoot up the limb, try *Hypericum perforatum* as above.

HERBAL REMEDIES
- Calendula ointment acts as an antiseptic on minor cuts and scrapes.
- Aloe gel is soothing and may help the healing process for minor wounds.

AROMATHERAPY
Tea tree oil is antiseptic. Add a few drops to water and wash the cut or scrape with it.

INSECT BITES & STINGS

SYMPTOMS

- Itching and soreness
- Red swollen bumps

ANAPHYLACTIC SHOCK:
- Swelling around the face, lips, or throat
- Difficulty breathing
- Severe itching, numbness, or cramps
- A rash
- Dizziness, faintness, loss of consciousness

Warning!
If someone stung by a bee or wasp has the symptoms of anaphylactic shock (see above), call 911. If the sting is in the mouth, get medical help immediately.

Insect bites are tiny wounds in the skin made by insects so they can suck blood. Insects inject venom into the skin to make this process easier.

CAUSES

- Insects that bite include mosquitoes, gnats, lice, blackflies, horseflies, sandflies, fleas, and bedbugs. Ticks, spiders, and mites, which are not insects but creatures known as arachnids, can also bite. In tropical areas, mosquito bites can cause malaria.
- Stings are usually from bees, wasps, and hornets. An allergic reaction to a bite or sting can cause life-threatening anaphylactic shock (see p.30–31.)

WHAT YOUR DOCTOR WOULD DO

You can treat most bites and stings at home. Wash the area thoroughly with soap and water. Apply a soothing lotion such as calamine. Avoid scratching the area. If it gets worse, see your doctor, who may prescribe an antihistamine.

If a bee's sting remains in the wound, gently scrape it out with a clean needle, or tweezers. Do not squeeze the sting, you may release more venom. Then wash carefully with soap and water and apply a cold compress.

If you have an allergic reaction to bee or wasp stings, you may need an injection of a drug called epinephrine.

4

ALTERNATIVE TREATMENTS

HERBAL REMEDIES

To relieve a sting, place a slice of onion or a fresh marigold flower, crushed, directly on the sting and bandage it in place.

Place a freshly sliced onion directly on a sting.

HOMEOPATHY

Ledum palustre is the classic remedy for simple bug bites. Take 2 pellets of 12c every two hours

---

LYME DISEASE

A tick that lives on deer in the United States and Europe can cause Lyme disease, a sometimes serious infection. One noticeable symptom is a bull's eye rash, but this is not always present. Other symptoms include headaches, fatigue, fever, chills, sore throat, and aches—all flulike symptoms. If caught early, doctors can treat it with antibiotics. If left untreated, it can cause arthritis or heart trouble. Prevention includes wearing pants tucked into socks and long-sleeved shirts in certain areas in the summer months. Also, use an insect repellent that contains DEET.

HIVES

- Extremely itchy rash with white blotches on red patches of skin

CALL A DOCTOR IF

- Hives develop in your throat
- You have hives for a month or longer

Warning!

If someone who has been stung or bitten develops hives, experiences dizziness and has difficulty in breathing, call 911 right away! The person may be suffering from a serious condition known as anaphylactic shock.

A skin reaction, or rash, from an allergy is known as hives. This can occur when the immune system overreacts to what it thinks is dangerous to the body. Hives usually disappear in a few hours, but can last for a few days, depending on the cause.

CAUSES

- Some types of foods can cause hives: the most common are milk, wheat, corn, citrus fruit, eggs, strawberries, and seafood.
- Certain medications, such as antibiotics and aspirin, can produce hives.
- Insect bites or stings or contact with a stinging plant, can cause hives.
- Hives can occur with exposure to heat, cold, sunlight, or after vigorous exertion.
- Emotional upsets and stress may also cause hives.

WHAT YOUR DOCTOR WOULD DO

Hives usually disappears on their own, but in the short term you can apply a soothing lotion such as calamine. If they don't go away after a couple of days or you get them often, see your doctor, who may prescribe an antihistamine drug or a cortisone ointment. Otherwise, try to work out what has caused the problem so you can avoid it in the future.

4

ALTERNATIVE TREATMENTS

HOMEOPATHY

For hives that result from getting chilled, as in cold air, try *Rhus toxicodendron* first—2 pellets of 30c under the tongue to repeat in 30 minutes as needed up to 6 doses.

HERBAL REMEDIES

A fresh cabbage leaf has anti-inflammatory properties. Place it directly on the hives. Or remove the centre rib of the leaf, then crush the leaf, and place it on the hives; apply a bandage to hold it in place.

Apply a cabbage leaf to the affected area.

ACUPRESSURE

To fortify the immune system, apply firm pressure with your thumb on top of your forearm, 2 thumbs' width above the wrist, for 1 minute. Repeat on the other arm.

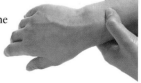

Acupressure point on the forearm

SHINGLES

- Pain or itching, usually on one side of the body or face, followed by:
- A strip or group of painful blisters
- A burning sensation at the site of the blisters
- Fever
- Generally feeling unwell

CALL A DOCTOR IF

- The rash appears near an eye
- A yellow crust forms, indicating bacterial infection
- You cannot bear the pain

In people who have had chicken pox, the virus that caused it, the herpes zoster virus, usually remains in the body but is dormant—it does not cause any problems. In some people the virus becomes active again at a later date, resulting in shingles.

Shingles typically occurs in elderly people, but can also appear in young people. Symptoms last for weeks or months, or, at worst, years. Shingles usually happens only once, but it has been known to recur in some people.

CAUSES

- Illness, injury, or emotional stress weakens the immune system, which can allow the virus to become active.

WHAT YOUR DOCTOR WOULD DO

Conventional medicine offers no cure, but the doctor will prescribe medicine to help reduce the pain and inflammation, and an antiviral drug to control the rash. Early treatment can decrease the intensity and duration of the rash and help prevent the pain that sometimes persists after the rash goes away. If the area becomes infected, you may need antibiotics.

4

ALTERNATIVE TREATMENTS

HOMEOPATHY

- Very itchy shingles better from warm baths or hot packs may respond to *Arsenicum album* or *Rhus toxicodendron* in 12 or 30c potencies, 2 pellets under the tongue every 2-4 hours as needed, up to 6 doses.
- For pain that persists after shingles are all gone, one remedy to try is *Kalmia latifolia*, or mountain laurel, dosed as above.

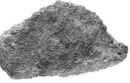

Arsenopyrite is the source for *Arsenicum album*.

HERBAL REMEDIES

- A solution of lemon balm or calendula can be gently applied to the affected area to reduce inflammation. To make a solution, first make a tincture: half-fill a large jar with the herb and fill with an alcohol (vodka is ideal). Cover and leave in a cool dark place. Shake twice a day for 2 weeks; then strain into another jar. Mix together 1 part tincture and 1 part boiled and cooled water. The solution is now ready to be used.
- A commercial gel containing licorice may help ease the pain of shingles.
- Skin preparations containing St John's wort (hypericum) are often effective.

BLISTERS & CHILBLAINS

BLISTERS:
- Bubblelike pockets in the skin filled with fluid; there may be one or many
- Sometimes pain, inflammation, or itching

CHILBLAINS:
- Itchy, purple-red swellings

CALL A DOCTOR IF

- The blister results from a chemical burn
- Blistering is caused by a serious case of sunburn
- If there is a discharge of pus

When the skin is irritated, bubblelike blisters can form. These may be the size of a pin prick or up to ½ inch (1 cm) in diameter or even more.

Chilblains are swellings that are usually found on the toes or fingers, although they may also develop on the nose and ears.

CAUSES
- Brief intense rubbing of the skin can cause contact blisters. Wearing new shoes or shoes that don't fit properly can cause blisters on the feet. Working with a handheld tool can create a blister on the palm.
- Burns and sunburn can cause blisters, as can certain chemicals.
- Blisters may also be a symptom of an illness, such as shingles, or a reaction to a drug such as penicillin.
- Chilblains are caused by the blood vessels narrowing too much in cold weather.

WHAT YOUR DOCTOR WOULD DO
Most blisters heal on their own. Because the fluid in a blister is sterile, it makes an excellent wound dressing if left intact. However, if you feel you have to pop it with a needle, sterilize the needle first by placing it in a flame or dipping it in an antiseptic solution.

Chilblains don't require treatment, although some people find applying unperfumed talcum powder to the area helps relieve the itching.

4

ALTERNATIVE TREATMENTS

 HOMEOPATHY
The burning, smarting pain of a recent burn may often be eased by taking *Cantharis* in a 6 or 12c potency, 2 pellets under the tongue every 2 hours as needed up to 12 doses.

 HERBAL REMEDIES
- Aloe vera gel may be rubbed onto a blister from a burn.
- For an antiseptic, mix 2 drops of chamomile oil in ½ cup (120 ml) of water. Apply to the blister; cover with a dressing.

 AROMATHERAPY
Dab a little lavender oil on the blister.

 REFLEXOLOGY
If you have chilblains, you can improve your circulation by working on this reflexology point. Apply pressure to the heart point on the left foot, just to the side of the ball of the foot.

Reflexology point to the side of the ball of the foot

SUNBURN

SYMPTOMS

- The skin turns red and feels hot and painful
- Dehydration
- Fever and chills
- Blisters may occur in severe cases, as well as nausea
- After a few days the skin will turn tan or brown colored and may peel

CALL A DOCTOR IF

- You have blisters, fever, and nausea

Warning!
Frequent sunburn, especially in childhood, can lead to skin cancer

The skin burns when it is overexposed to ultraviolet rays from the sun. Light-skinned people are most vulnerable, but dark-skinned people can burn, too. Sunburn usually appears 1 to 6 hours after overexposure to the sun.

CAUSES
- Exposure to direct sunlight puts you at risk of sunburn. The severity of the burn depends on how long you stay in the sun and where you are. Burning occurs more rapidly at higher altitudes and toward the equator and can sometimes take place after only 15 minutes in the sun.
- Sunlight reflected from sand, water, or snow is just as strong as direct sunlight.
- Some medicines, such as certain prescriptions to treat acne, make the skin extra-sensitive to sunlight.

WHAT YOUR DOCTOR WOULD DO
For mild sunburn, apply a soothing lotion, such as calamine or a preparation containing aloe vera, and wait for the discomfort to die down. It's important to drink plenty and to avoid further sun exposure. For severe sunburn, the doctor may prescribe drugs to ease the pain. Hospitalization is necessary in extreme cases.

4

ALTERNATIVE TREATMENTS

HOMEOPATHY
- For dry, hot, crimson skin, tender to the slightest touch or bump, try *Belladonna* 30c, 2 pellets every hour up to 6 doses.

Coneflower is the source of echinacea.

HERBAL REMEDIES
A cold compress soaked in a calendula infusion is soothing; steep 1 teaspoon of the dried herb in a cup of boiling water for 10 minutes. Or use an echinacea infusion on blistering skin to prevent infection.

AVOIDING SUNBURN

- Stay out of the sun if you can when it is at its strongest—between 10:00 a.m. and 3:00 p.m., especially in summer. If your shadow is shorter than your height, the sun is strong.
- When outside, wear loose clothes that cover and protect your arms and legs, and a wide-brimmed hat to protect your face.
- Use sunscreen or block on exposed skin. Make sure the sunscreen's sun protection factor (SPF) is at least 15. Remember to reapply it as necessary.
- Protect your eyes with sunglasses that give UV protection.

ACNE

- Recurrent red swellings, or pimples, on the skin, usually on the face, neck, back, shoulders, and chest
- Dark pores, known as blackheads
- Infected, pus-filled pimples
- Scarring may occur

CYST:
- Hard, inflamed swelling in the skin
- Occasionally infection
- Scarring may occur

CAUSES

- Acne is most common in the teenage years, particularly in boys, and is caused by an over-sensitivity to normal amounts of the hormone testosterone, present in males and females.
- People with oily skin are more likely to have acne.
- About one in five adults has acne. Women are more likely to have pimples continuing into their 30s; these are usually more likely before a period.
- A woman may have a flare-up just before she reaches menopause.
- Heredity may play a part.
- The contraceptive Pill can trigger acne, though one particular type reduces it.
- Other medicines, such as corticocsteroids, can cause acne.
- A poor diet can aggravate acne; but only a very few people find that any particular foods make their acne worse.
- Stress and lack of sleep can make acne worse.
- A type of acne can occur in newborns and infants, particularly in boys. It appears on the face and clears up within weeks, leaving no lasting marks.
- A cyst develops when a spot becomes infected and the infection goes deep into the skin. ▶

4

ALTERNATIVE TREATMENTS

HOMEOPATHY

- For acne along the jaw line in teenage girls who crave salt and shun company, consider *Natrum muriaticum*, 12c daily for a month or two.
- For acne right on the tip of the nose, *Causticum* in a 12 or 30c potency, 2 pellets under the tongue daily for up to a week, may prove very helpful.

Sulfur, the source of *Hepar sulfuris*, for treating pimples

HERBAL REMEDIES

- A facial steam bath with fresh chamomile flowers or sage leaves can help open up pores. Making sure that

Facial steam bath with chamomile flowers can open up pores.

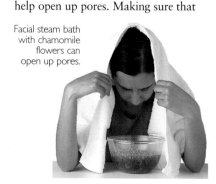

WHAT YOUR DOCTOR WOULD DO
Many different treatments may help, including applications of creams and lotions that can unblock the pores and promote healing. You can buy over-the-counter treatments for pimples or minor acne. Your doctor may prescribe drugs such as antibiotics, the contraceptive Pill (for girls only) or vitamin-A derivatives called retinoids in more severe cases.

CALL A DOCTOR IF

- After using over-the-counter medicines for 2–3 months, the pimples or blackheads don't clear up
- Infection develops in pimples or cysts

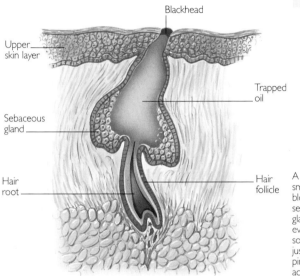

Blackhead

Upper skin layer

Trapped oil

Sebaceous gland

Hair root

Hair follicle

A pimple develops when a small hair follicle becomes blocked by an oily secretion from a sebaceous gland in the skin. Just about everyone has pimples at some time. There may be just a few scattered pimples or much more acne over a large area.

4

ALTERNATIVE TREATMENTS

the water isn't scalding, bend your head over a bowl of hot water containing a handful of the herb of your choice, for no more than 15 minutes. Hold a towel over your head to trap the steam.
- Try a skin wash to reduce infection and inflammation. Using one of the following strained preparations, dab it gently on the affected area with surgical cotton: a teaspoon of tincture of calendula (from a health food store) mixed with a cup of water; a chamomile tea bag steeped in a cup of covered water for 10 minutes; a handful of fresh or dried yarrow, elder, or lavender steeped in water for 10 minutes.

ACUPRESSURE
To ease inflammation, bend your left elbow and press your thumb on the outer edge of the elbow crease for 1 minute; repeat on the other side.

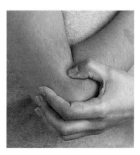

Acupressure point near the elbow, on the outer edge of the crease

DERMATITIS & ECZEMA

SYMPTOMS

DERMATITIS:
- Red, itchy skin
- Scales or, in acute attacks, oozing blisters

CONTACT DERMATITIS:
- A red rash where the skin has come in contact with an irritant

SEBORRHEIC DERMATITIS:
- Yellowish greasy scales on the scalp, behind the ears, around the nose, and on the eyebrows

ECZEMA:
- Dry, itchy skin
- Thick patches on the wrists, face, and creases of the elbows and knees
- Blisters and, later, scaling

Dermatitis is a broad term for skin inflammation and includes contact dermatitis, seborrheic dermatitis, and eczema.

CAUSES

- Contact dermatitis has many possible causes. Among them are some plants, such as poison ivy, poison oak, and certain garden plants; some fruits and vegetables, including oranges; household chemicals such as detergents, soaps, and nail polish remover; and cosmetics and skin-care products.
- Wearing jewelry containing nickel, rubber gloves, and new clothes before they have been washed can also cause contact dermatitis.
- Seborrheic dermatitis can lead to dandruff or, in babies, cradle cap. The cause is unknown but stress can aggravate it.
- Eczema is often associated with an allergy. The chief culprits are cows' milk, eggs, wheat, nuts, house dust mites, pollen, wool, detergents, and nickel in jewelry, cutlery, and zippers. Stress can also be a trigger. Eczema often runs in families, and other family members may suffer from asthma or allergic rhinitis (hay fever). ▶

4

ALTERNATIVE TREATMENTS

 HERBAL REMEDIES
Do not use any of these herbs for more than a month without consulting a trained herbalist.
- Infusions of dandelion or burdock can help eczema. Brew a tablespoon of the grated dried root in a cup of boiling water for 10 minutes and strain before drinking. Drink 3 cups a day.
- Evening primrose oil can help many people with hereditary eczema.

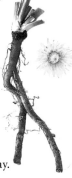

The root of the dandelion can relieve eczema.

For an adult, take up to 6 capsules a day. **Warning!** Do not use evening primrose oil if you are pregnant, have high cholesterol, or have liver disease.

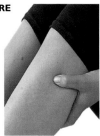 **ACUPRESSURE**
Exert pressure for 1 minute on a point 4 finger's width below the knee to relieve stress and strengthen the immune system.

Acupressure point below the knee

WHAT YOUR DOCTOR WOULD DO

Treatments are aimed at soothing the skin. For mild cases, a bath followed by an application of an over-the-counter cream containing hydrocortisone is the first step. Your doctor may prescribe antihistamines, which combat allergic reactions, or antibiotics for an infection.

If contact dermatitis is suspected, or if it is thought that eczema is caused by an allergy, it is important to find the trigger—whatever it is that you are allergic to. Your doctor can do this by applying various irritants to your skin to see whether there is any reaction. One way to avoid some hand eczema is to wear white cotton gloves under rubber gloves when doing housework.

Antibiotics may be prescribed for severe cases of eczema.

Moisturizing your skin helps many types of eczema. Unperfumed bath oil might help keep the skin moist. It is also important to avoid scratching your skin, as this only makes the rash worse and can lead to infection.

CALL A DOCTOR IF

- There are signs of a skin infection, such as oozing pus
- The condition doesn't respond to over-the-counter medicines
- The sufferer is a baby less than 18 months old
- You have eczema and come into contact with someone who has a viral infection of the skin, such as cold sores or warts

4

REFLEXOLOGY

To treat eczema, a reflexologist concentrates on points which treat either the skin condition itself or the body as a whole. The point just below the bottom of the big toenail is suitable if the face is affected by dermatitis. The reflexology point for the adrenals, which can help reduce inflammation and allergy,

is located just below the ball of the foot.

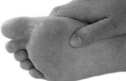

Adrenals point just below the ball of the foot

Face point at the bottom of big toenail

AROMATHERAPY

Creams or nutrients containing essential oils of lavender or chamomile help reduce inflammation in some people with eczema.

PSORIASIS

4

SYMPTOMS

- Red and inflamed itchy skin, usually with whitish silvery scales; in particular, on the scalp, elbows, and knees, although it can occur anywhere on the body
- Discoloration, thickening, and pitting of the fingernails and toenails; the nails may pull away from the underlying nailbed

CALL A DOCTOR IF

- The condition worsens while taking a prescribed medication or the problem persists

Psoriasis is a common skin complaint that occurs when skin cell production is abnormally high— about 10 times higher than average. This huge number of cells forms into white scaly patches, which can be uncomfortable and embarrassing. Psoriasis is rare in people with dark skin and usually appears between the ages of 10 and 40, although it can develop in babies and older people too.

CAUSES

- The cause is unknown, although psoriasis sometimes runs in families.
- Psoriasis may be triggered by illness, such as a streptococcal throat infection, stress, certain medicines, or obesity.

WHAT YOUR DOCTOR WOULD DO

There is no known cure for psoriasis, but good treatment can keep most attacks under control. For mild psoriasis, your doctor may recommend taking a warm bath for 15 minutes to remove the scaly skin, then applying a preparation which helps the skin retain moisture. Certain drugs may help, including creams that promote the shedding of the scales and an ointment that prevents inflammation. In severe cases, the doctor may suggest steroid drugs or therapy in which drugs are taken and the skin is exposed to ultraviolet radiation.

ALTERNATIVE TREATMENTS

HERBAL REMEDIES

- Try an infusion of dandelion or burdock root or Oregon grape. Steep 1 tablespoon of the dried herb in a cup of boiling water for 10 minutes and strain. You can drink up to 3 cups daily.
- If the psoriasis is on the scalp, try a daily hair rinse containing dried rosemary and sage. Steep 1 ounce (25 g) of each herb in a 1 pint (500 ml) of boiling water. Let it stand overnight. Strain it, and use after shampooing.

AROMATHERAPY

- Mix 4 drops of the essential oil of juniper and 2 drops of cedarwood with a 1 tablespoon of almond or olive oil. Three times a week, cover your scalp with the mixture and cover with a shower cap overnight. Wash out the next morning. **Warning!** Do not use juniper or cedarwood oils if pregnant.

Juniper is used to make an essential oil that can help psoriasis.

CORNS & CALLUSES

SYMPTOMS

- An uncomfortable, sometimes painful, area of thick, dead skin on the feet or elsewhere

CALL A DOCTOR IF

- The corn or callus discharges pus or a clear fluid—it may be infected
- You suffer from diabetes, or any other condition causing poor circulation

Both calluses and corns are thickened areas of dead skin that form to protect underlying tissues. A callus is common on the palm, fingers, and the ball of the foot or the heel. Constant pressure and friction on the skin can result in a corn on a toe.

CAUSES

- Corns and calluses may be due to ill-fitting shoes.
- Walking incorrectly can also cause them.
- People with physically demanding manual jobs may develop calluses on their hands.
- Musicians who play a stringed instrument, such as the violin, viola, cello, or guitar, sometimes have calluses on the tips of their fingers.

WHAT A DOCTOR WOULD DO

A doctor may scrape off some of the skin to determine if you have a callus or a wart—a wart will bleed. A corn or callus will go away by itself once you avoid the friction or pressure responsible; but if it bothers you, it can be cut away by a doctor or chiropodist—a specialist in treating feet.

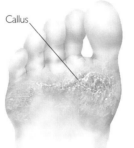

Callus

Corn

4

ALTERNATIVE TREATMENTS

HERBAL REMEDIES

- Apply a little calendula cream to the corn or callus to soften it.
- Crush a clove of garlic and hold it against the corn with a bandage to protect and soften the affected area.

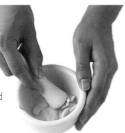

Crush the garlic using a mortar and pestle or the flat side of the blade of a chef's knife.

AVOIDING CORNS

- Wearing shoes that fit properly is the best way to avoid corns. Have your feet measured in the shoe store the next time you buy shoes to make sure you are getting shoes of the correct length and width.
- Don't wear high heels all day, every day. Try to alternate your shoes so that you wear a different pair of shoes each day during any 3-day period.
- If corns are caused by the way you walk or stand, try wearing a special insole in your shoes.

BOILS, CARBUNCLES, & WARTS

SYMPTOMS

BOIL:
■ An inflamed reddish sore, sometimes with a yellow or white center, that is painful and filled with pus

WART:
■ A small, raised bump of hard skin on the hand, knee, or face, or foot

WART HYGIENE

■ Don't share towels and face cloths if you have a wart
■ Wear a bandage on a plantar wart if swimming
■ Don't touch a wart or shave near it—you could spread it to other parts of the body

A boil occurs when a hair follicle or oil gland becomes infected. A cluster of boils is called a carbuncle. Boils are most likely on the face, the back of the neck, and the buttocks.

Warts are caused by a viral infection in the skin. A wart on the foot is called a plantar wart.

CAUSES
■ A bacterial infection that enters the skin through a hair follicle.
■ A contagious viral infection that causes warts. The virus can be spread by direct contact from the floor in moist environments, such as in showers and locker rooms or from shared bathmats or towels.

WHAT YOUR DOCTOR WOULD DO
Boils usually burst by themselves within a few days or weeks. If you have a carbuncle, see your doctor, or you may need a course of antibiotics to clear up the infection. Painful boils should be lanced only by a doctor to avoid the risk of further infection.

Warts usually go away within a few months, but you can buy various over-the-counter treatments to help get rid of them. Because these contain harsh chemicals, they are not recommended for the face. If the wart doesn't go away, your doctor may burn it off using liquid nitrogen.

4

ALTERNATIVE TREATMENTS

HOMEOPATHY
■ For warts at the tips of the fingers, around the nails, or on the nose, try *Causticum* 12c, 2 pellets daily under the tongue, for 1 month. Do not use concurrently with tea tree oil, which will antidote its effectiveness.

HERBAL REMEDIES
■ Compresses made with comfrey, slippery elm, or burdock infusions can help a boil come to a head. First make an infusion by steeping 1 or 2 teaspoons of any of these dried herbs in a cup of boiling water for 10 minutes. Soak a

clean cloth in the infusion, wring it out, and apply it to the boil.
■ To fight off the virus, bathe a wart in tea tree oil or the juice from a dandelion stem.
■ Apply a crushed garlic clove or slice of onion to a wart. Hold it in place with a bandage.

Chop a garlic clove, then crush it before use.

ATHLETE'S FOOT & RINGWORM

ATHLETE'S FOOT:
- An itchy red rash that may crack and peel, usually between the toes but sometimes on the sole of the foot
- Unpleasant foot odor
- Toenails that are brittle and flaky

RINGWORM:
- A small red patch that grows into an itchy, ring-shaped rash

CALL A DOCTOR IF

- Athlete's foot does not respond to over-the-counter medicines after a month or if the skin becomes swollen or weepy

Athlete's foot is a fungal infection of the feet that thrives in warm, moist environments and feeds on a protein in skin, nails, and hair.

Ringworm is a fungal infection. It is not caused by a worm at all—the name is descriptive of the appearance of some rashes. It can be found in the groin and on the feet, scalp, nails, and torso and is most common in children.

CAUSES
- As the name suggests, athlete's foot is common among athletes, who wear airtight training shoes that provide the ideal conditions for the fungus to grow. It can also be picked up from skin particles shed in shoes and towels and on shower floors and around swimming pools.
- Ringworm is a contagious disease that spreads from infected people and domestic animals.

WHAT YOUR DOCTOR WOULD DO
Athlete's foot sometimes clears up by itself; or, antifungal powders and creams that you can buy over the counter usually work. The most important advice is to keep the feet clean and dry, air them as much as you can, and wear clean socks. In severe cases, the doctor may prescribe antifungal drugs. Antifungal cream or drugs may also be prescribed for ringworm.

4

ALTERNATIVE TREATMENTS

 HERBAL REMEDIES
Tea tree oil can help ringworm or athlete's foot: rub it on the affected area daily.

AROMATHERAPY
For athlete's foot, soak your feet in a bowl of warm water with a few drops of tea tree oil.

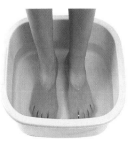

A foot bath with tea tree oil is helpful for athlete's foot.

SCABIES

Scabies is caused by an infestation with a tiny mite that enters the skin and lays eggs. It is usually found between the fingers, on the wrists, and on the genitals. It causes gray scaly swellings and is extremely itchy and infectious.

Your doctor will prescribe a lotion to kill the mites. Because they spread rapidly, everyone in your home should use it, even if they have no symptoms.

Wash all recently used clothes, linens, and towels in hot water. Clean all your tables, chairs, floors, and carpets. Keep difficult-to-clean items, like stuffed toys, sealed in storage for a week.

DANDRUFF & LICE

SYMPTOMS

DANDRUFF:
- White flakes of skin on the scalp, often falling onto the shoulders

LICE:
- Itchy red spots in the affected area.

CALL A DOCTOR IF

- You have scalp irritation and thick scales despite regular use of antidandruff shampoos
- You have yellowish crusting and red patches along the neckline—this may be seborrheic dandruff, which requires treatment with presciption drugs

Dandruff is a condition in which dead skin flakes off, noticeably from the scalp; it is usually little problem, although a bit embarrassing.

Lice are tiny insects that feed on the blood and leave eggs and small, itchy bites. There are three types, and they are all contagious: head lice live on the scalp; body lice live on the clothes and visit the body to feed; and pubic lice live in the pubic hair and are also known as "crabs."

CAUSES
- Dandruff can result from sebaceous glands producing too much oil, or from a fungal infection.
- Dermatitis (see pp.66–67) or psoriasis (see p.68) can cause dandruff.
- Lice spread when people are in close contact.

WHAT YOUR DOCTOR WOULD DO
Washing your hair with medicated shampoos usually clears up dandruff. In severe cases, your doctor may prescribe corticosteroid cream.

Head lice are best treated with twice weekly shampooing for two weeks; each time, condition well to get rid of the tangles. Then rinse and comb well with a fine-toothed comb. This should help you avoid insecticidal lotion or shampoos. Body lice and pubic lice require insecticidal lotions. For pubic lice, sexual partners should be treated at the same time.

4

ALTERNATIVE TREATMENTS

 HERBAL REMEDIES
- Both thyme and rosemary are effective remedies. Boil 2 heaping teaspoons of one of the herbs in a cup of water for 10 minutes, strain, and cool. Massage the liquid into your scalp. Do not rinse it off.
- Massage tea tree oil into your scalp to help prevent infection. Keep the oil away from your eyes.

AROMATHERAPY
Use the essential oils of rosemary and red thyme to treat head lice. Mix 6 drops of each in 2 cups (500 ml) of warm water; use as a hair rinse after shampooing.

HEAD LICE HYGIENE

- Wash all clothes, towels, and linens that may have been used by an infected person in hot soapy water and dry in a hot dryer. Soak combs, brushes, and other hair items in hot soapy water for 10 minutes. Or place infected items in sealed plastic bags for 2 weeks. The eggs will hatch and die of starvation.
- Treat all the members of the family at once.
- To avoid spreading head lice, do not send an infected child to school until after the lice have been treated. Inform the school of the problem.

Women's Health

Children's Health

WOMEN'S HEALTH

Women have special health issues that are often related to their reproductive system. These can be a minor inconvenience, such as a craving for a certain food during menstruation, or may have a signifcant effect on a woman's health such as the loss of calcium in the bones that can occur in menopause.

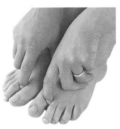

CHILDREN'S HEALTH

Babies and young children are susceptible to certain ailments that do not affect them when they are older, for example, diaper rash and colic. This is the time when they receive most of their vaccinations, which have reduced the risk of many childhood diseases, such as mumps, measles, hepatitis, and meningitis.

5

BLADDER INFECTIONS

SYMPTOMS

- A burning sensation when urinating.
- A frequent need to urinate
- A feeling that the bladder still needs to be emptied after you have been to the toilet
- Strong odor from the urine

CALL A DOCTOR IF

- Cystitis does not clear up by itself within 24 hours
- You have a fever, vomiting, blood in the urine, or back or abdominal pain
- The burning sensation is accompanied by a discharge from the vagina or penis

An infection caused by bacteria that normally live in the intestines can lead to inflammation of the bladder, known as cystitis. Bladder infections are more common in women because they have a shorter urine passage, or urethra, which conveys urine from the bladder, than men do.

CAUSES

- Sexual intercourse can cause a bladder infection by pushing the bacteria up the urethra into the bladder. In some women, this happens every time they have sex.
- An infection can occur when a diaphragm is used for birth control. The bladder does not always empty completely when the device is in place, and the stagnant urine encourages bacteria to multiply.
- Pregnant women may get bladder infections because of the pressure of the baby on the bladder.

WHAT YOUR DOCTOR WOULD DO

If a bladder infection doesn't clear up in a day after trying a remedy below, see your doctor, who may prescribe antibiotics after giving you a urine test.

Preventive measures include drinking at least 4 pints (2 liters) of water a day, not holding your bladder for long periods of time, wiping from front to back after using the toilet, urinating after sex, and not using vaginal douches or deodorants.

ALTERNATIVE TREATMENTS

HOMEOPATHY

- For burning pain during urination, try *Cantharis* in a 6 or 12c potency, 2 pellets under the tongue before every urination until better, or up to 6 times.
- For pain at the end of urination, as your muscles squeeze closed, try *Sarsaparilla* in the same way.
- For bladder infections in women that follow intercourse, *Staphysagria* again dosed as above, is often a good choice.

HERBAL REMEDIES

- Cranberry juice fights the bacteria that can cause a bladder infection. Drink up

to 16 fluid ounces (500 ml) a day to get rid of an infection. Try to find a preparation with a low sugar content, or use 2 capsules 4 times daily.

ACUPRESSURE

Apply pressure just above your pubic bone for 1 minute, then gently massage around the area.

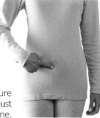

The acupressure point for cystitis is just above your pubic bone.

5

YEAST INFECTIONS (THRUSH)

SYMPTOMS

- Soreness and itching of the vagina and redness and swelling in the area
- A vaginal discharge that resembles cottage cheese
- Pain during sexual intercourse

CALL A DOCTOR IF

- You are uncertain whether you have a yeast infection
- Your symptoms do not disappear after a week of treatment with appropriate over-the-counter preparations

A yeast infection is caused by the fungus *Candida albicans*. It usually occurs in the vagina. It is possible to get yeast infections in other moist areas of the body, such as in the mouth, in which case it is known as thrush.

CAUSES

- It can be triggered by being generally fatigued, or sometimes by taking antibiotics.
- Diabetics are more likely to develop yeast infections because the high levels of sugar in their blood and urine encourage yeasts to grow.
- Although yeast infections can be passed on sexually, it is common to get it without ever having had sex.

WHAT YOUR DOCTOR WOULD DO

Effective treatments for yeast infections and thrush are available over-the-counter in the form of anti-fungal creams ot tablets. Yeast infections often have no symptoms in men even when there is an infection, so ask your sexual partner to apply the cream to the head of his penis to avoid having the problem passed straight back to you.

In stubborn cases, your doctor may prescribe anti-fungal drugs.

ALTERNATIVE TREATMENTS

HERBAL REMEDIES
- A calendula infusion can help. Steep 1 or 2 teaspoons of the dried herb in a cup of boiling water and strain. Use as a douche when cool.
- An over-the-counter ointment containing chickweed can relieve itchiness.

Chickweed in an ointment eases irritation.

SELF-HELP STEPS

- Eat a healthy diet
- Eating live plain yogurt may help replace the bacteria that can guard against yeast infections. Putting yogurt directly in the vagina may be soothing.
- After you have used the toilet, always wipe from front to back.
- Avoid using perfumed products around the vagina, and don't put them in the bath. Don't use douches or vaginal deodorants.
- Wear white cotton underpants, which allow air to circulate. Avoid wearing clothes made of synthetic fibers, which increase moistness.

5

PREMENSTRUAL SYNDROME (PMS)

SYMPTOMS

- Irritability and anxiety
- Feeling tearful and depressed
- Abdominal bloating and tenderness
- Swollen, tender breasts
- Headaches
- Water retention
- Weight gain, up to 5 pounds (2.25 kg)
- Back and muscle aches
- Abdominal pain
- Fatigue or drowsiness
- Excess energy
- Nausea
- Diarrhea or constipation
- Breaking out in pimples or cold sores
- Craving for sugary or salty foods or for chocolate

Premenstrual syndrome, or PMS, is the name given to a range of symptoms that many women experience a few days to a week before a period. The symptoms vary: some women have only one minor symptom while others have a dozen or so. Sometimes the symptoms are so severe that a woman has to seek help from her doctor.

Causes

- No one knows precisely what causes PMS. In fact, the medical profession often disagrees about suspected causes. There are many theories that may account for some of the symptoms.
- An imbalance in certain hormone levels can cause symptoms.
- A fluctuation in brain chemicals can trigger premenstrual syndrome.
- Dietary deficiencies, such as insufficient vitamin B_6, may be responsible for some symptoms, including fluid retention and bloating, tender breasts, and fatigue. Stress can reduce the level of magnesium in the body, which is perhaps why some women crave food high in magnesium, such as chocolate. Low levels of essential fatty acids may affect mood.
- Premenstrual syndrome may have a genetic cause. Identical twins are more likely to suffer the same symptoms than fraternal twins. ▶

ALTERNATIVE TREATMENTS

AROMATHERAPY
- Place a drop of the essential oil of Roman chamomile or melissa on a handkerchief and inhale the scent.
- Add a few drops of the essential oils of geranium, clary sage, and lavender to a bath for 2 weeks before your period.

Roman chamomile can help relieve PMS.

HOMEOPATHY
Try *Pulsatilla* 30c for tearfulness and *Sepia* 30c

for tender breasts, pain, and mood swings. Take in the morning or evening a day before symptoms are due.

ACUPRESSURE
Press your thumb on the inside of your leg 4 fingers' width above the ankle for 1 minute; repeat on the other leg. **Warning!** Do not do if you are pregnant.

Acupressure point above the ankle

5

WHAT YOUR DOCTOR WOULD DO

Your doctor may prescribe certain antidepressants to help reduce mood swings if they are severe. Some doctors may recommend taking certain hormones, perhaps in the form of injections or suppositories (tablets inserted into the vagina). Taking the contraceptive Pill or diuretic drugs to reduce water retention, can help reduce symptoms in some women. These methods, however, are not always helpful and may have undesirable side effects.

Evening primrose oil is rapidly gaining acceptance as a way to increase low levels of essential fatty acids.

CALL A DOCTOR IF

■ Your symptoms are so severe that you cannot cope with your daily routine

HERBAL REMEDIES

■ Dandelion leaves may help reduce bloating and swollen breasts. Skullcap can help alleviate irritability. Make an infusion of either of these herbs by steeping a tablespoon of the dried herb in a cup of boiling water for 10 minutes.
■ St John's wort may help depression. Try a 300-mg capsule 2–3 times per day.
■ Evening primrose oil has been found to be helpful for breast tenderness. Try 2 perles (capsules) twice daily.
■ Some women find taking 100–200 mg of vitamin B6 in combination with 500–1,000 mg of magnesium once or twice a day helpful

SELF HELP FOR PMS

■ Eat a healthy diet full of fruits, vegetables, and whole grains. Limit fats and sweets, reduce salt.
■ Instead of having 3 main meals a day, eat small meals every 3 hours. One theory suggests that low blood sugar causes PMS symptoms.
■ Eliminating tobacco and alcohol may relieve some symptoms. Avoiding caffeine helps decrease breast tenderness.
■ Regular exercise decreases PMS symptoms.
■ Reduce stress—try yoga or breathing exercises and get plenty of sleep.

5

MENSTRUAL CRAMPS

SYMPTOMS

- Menstruation may be painful at the beginning of the period and for up to 1 or 2 days
- Blood clots in the discharge

CALL A DOCTOR IF

- You have a menstrual flow that is so heavy that tampons have to be changed within an hour
- You have sharp pain before your period starts or during sexual intercourse

Most women have painful periods at some time in their lives, usually between the ages of 17 and 25. This condition is known as dysmenorrhea. It is often not as painful once a women has had a child.

CAUSES

- The pain is probably caused by the body producing too much of a particular prostaglandin, a hormonelike substance that makes the womb contract, in much the same way that it does during childbirth. Tightenings of the womb cause the muscle cramps.

WHAT YOUR DOCTOR WOULD DO

Period pains are usually simply an unpleasant inconvenience that can be relieved with over-the-counter anti-inflammatory painkillers. But if the cramps are very bad and stop you from carrying out your daily routine for long, you should see your doctor, who may examine you to rule out a more serious problem. Your doctor may recommend you to take the contraceptive Pill or prescribe stronger anti-inflammatory type pain pills.

ALTERNATIVE TREATMENTS

HERBAL REMEDIES

Cramp bark and chamomile flowers can help reduce period cramps. Steep 3 teaspoons of the dried herb in a cup of boiling water for about 15 minutes. Drink up to 3 times a day.

AROMATHERAPY

The essential oils of cajuput, sage, aniseed, cypress, and marjoram are all recommended for painful periods. Mix a few drops of one of these oils with a tablespoon of a base oil, such as almond or soybean. Starting 10 days before your period is due, gently massage the mixture over your abdomen and lower back each day.

ACUPRESSURE

Using your index fingers, press into the spaces between the big and second toes, angling the fingers slightly toward the second toe, and rub firmly before applying pressure for 1 minute.

Acupressure point between the big and second toe

5

HEAVY PERIODS

Most women lose about 2 ounces (60 ml) of blood during menstruation, but with heavy periods, known as menorrhagia, 3 ounces (90 ml) or more can be lost.

CAUSES

- An imbalance of certain hormones may be to blame because they may cause the lining of the womb to build up excessively.
- A disorder of the uterus, such as a fibroid, endometriosis, or a pelvic infection, may cause heavy periods. Using an IUD as a form of birth control may also cause heavy periods.

WHAT A DOCTOR WOULD DO

It's important to see the doctor to find the cause of the problem. Hormones and anti-inflammatory medications such as ibuprofen may be prescribed to decrease the flow. Iron tablets may also be recommended if you have iron-deficiency anemia.

If you still experience problems, your doctor may suggest an ultrasound examination of the pelvic organs, a biopsy of the inside of the uterus, or a simple operation known as a "D and C" (dilation and curettage), where the lining of the uterus is gently cleared out under general anesthetic. In the most severe cases, a hysterectomy (surgically removing the uterus) may be necessary.

ALTERNATIVE TREATMENTS

HERBAL REMEDIES

- Yarrow tea can control bleeding. Steep a teaspoon of the dried herb in a cup of boiling water for 10 minutes and strain. **Warning!** Do not take if you are pregnant.
- Shepherd's purse is used to regulate menstrual bleeding. You can make a tea by steeping a teaspoon of the dried herb in a cup of boiling water for 10 minutes, then straining it.

Yarrow used in a tea can reduce menstrual bleeding.

AROMATHERAPY

To provide relief from heavy periods, gently massage your abdomen in a clockwise motion with a few drops of the essential oils of cypress, geranium, and juniper mixed with a tablespoon of a base oil, such as almond or soybean.

Cypress, geranium, and juniper essential oils are beneficial for heavy periods.

5

PREGNANCY DISCOMFORTS

SYMPTOMS

MORNING SICKNESS:
- Feeling nauseus or vomiting, usually only until the 12th week of pregnancy. Bouts can occur in the morning or at any time of day

BACKACHE:
- Pain in the lower back that starts during the second trimester

HEARTBURN:
- Toward the end of pregnancy, an uncomfortable burning sensation in the upper abdomen, which is often worse at night

SORE BREASTS:
- The breasts feel tender and enlarged, almost from the start of pregnancy

Most pregnancies produce healthy babies at the end of nine months without any medical complications. During pregnancy, however, it is common for the expectant mother to experience a number of discomforts caused by the changes in her body. The most common complaints are morning sickness, back pain, heartburn, and sore breasts.

CAUSES

- One theory is that morning sickness is caused by a change in the hormone levels that occurs during pregnancy, which may trigger activity in the part of the brain that regulates vomiting.
- The increased weight of a growing unborn baby puts strain on the back.
- Heartburn is caused by acid reflux from upward pressure on the stomach as the uterus expands.
- Certain hormones prepare the breasts for breastfeeding by stimulating the development of the milk ducts and glands; these changes can cause a certain amount of soreness and irritation of the breasts. ▶

ALTERNATIVE TREATMENTS

HOMEOPATHY

Although the course of one's pregnancy, and ultimately labor and delivery, can be immeasurably enhanced by the appropriate use of Homeopathic medicines, it is such an important time that we would recommend seeking advice from experienced professionals, and not treating symptomatically.

HERBAL REMEDIES

To make an infusion, steep 1 or 2 teaspoons of one of the following herbs in a cup of boiling water for 10 minutes and strain if necessary.

- An infusion made from dried peppermint leaves may relieve morning sickness.
- An infusion of freshly grated ginger can also be effective.
- A chamomile flower or ginger infusion can help reduce heartburn when drunk after meals.

Grate root ginger to make an infusion..

AROMATHERAPY
- Add a few drops of the essential oils of lavender or geranium to warm bath water to help sore breasts.

5

WHAT YOUR DOCTOR WOULD DO

These problems won't normally require a doctor's attention, but certain self-help measures will make you feel more comfortable.

■ For morning sickness, eat small, frequent snacks instead of three large meals. Drink a lot of fluids, too.

■ To minimize backache, avoid putting on unnecessary weight: stick to a healthy diet and remember you don't have to "eat for two." Don't stand for long periods and avoid stretching up to reach higher places. Try to sit straight and make sure you have a firm mattress to sleep on. Bend your knees keeping your back straight when you have to lift something, and avoid lifting heavy items. Don't wear high-heeled shoes except for once in a while.

■ Eating little and often instead of three heavy meals can provide relief from heartburn. Try to avoid spicy or fatty foods. In bed, use extra pillows under your head so that your body is raised instead of flat, or raise the head of the bed 4 inches (10 cm) by safely propping up the legs. If the heartburn is extremely uncomfortable, your doctor may prescribe antacids or other drugs.

■ Sore breasts should be supported by the correct size bra throughout pregnancy. Pure lanolin rubbed onto nipples may help soreness and relieve dryness.

CALL A DOCTOR IF

■ You have severe nausea or vomiting
■ There is vaginal spotting or bleeding
■ You have a severe headache, blurred vision, sudden weight gain, or swollen fingers
■ Backache with fever
■ Blood in the urine
■ Once the baby moves, the movements decrease or stop for more than a day

Warning!
Consult your doctor or a licensed practitioner before trying an alternative therapy. Some remedies have adverse effects on pregnant women.

■ For morning sickness, add a few drops of the essential oils of chamomile or rose to a handkerchief and inhale the scent.

ACUPRESSURE

■ For morning sickness, place your thumb 2 fingers' widths above the crease of your wrist on the inside of the arm. Massage in a circular motion for 1 minute. Repeat on the other wrist.

■ Place your thumbs on your back, 1 inch (2.5 cm) on each side of the spine, just behind the navel, and press inward for 1 minute. Or rub the area with the back of your hands.

Acupressure point above the wrist

Acupressure points near the spine for back pain

5

MENOPAUSE

SYMPTOMS

- Periods may become lighter and more infrequent before stopping completely
- Periods may be unpredictable for a while, with varying degrees of heaviness
- Menstruation may stop suddenly
- You may experience hot flashes—a sudden intense feeling of heat that spreads over the face and neck. Hot flashes usually last only a few moments, but may occur many times during the day
- At night, hot flashes, accompanied by increased sweating may cause insomnia
- You may begin to experience vaginal dryness

Menopause is when a woman's periods stop altogether. This usually happens between the ages of 45 and 55, although it may occur sooner or later. When a woman reaches menopause, she may have an increased risk of certain medical problems.

CAUSES

- Levels of the female hormone estrogen decrease in the years leading up to menopause and can cause various symptoms which differ from person to person.
- The lower levels of estrogen may have an effect on the health of a woman's bones; in some women the bones become so thin and brittle that a painful condition called osteoporosis develops. Women who are thin and have a light bone structure are at a higher risk, as are women who smoke, are heavy drinkers, or live sedentary lives. Women who have had anorexia nervosa in the past have a higher risk of osteoporosis, too.
- Reduced levels of estrogen are a major contributing factor in the sharply increased risk of heart disease among post-menopausal women. ▶

ALTERNATIVE TREATMENTS

 AROMATHERAPY

To improve your physical well-being, relax in a bath after adding 5 drops of the essential oil of sage and 2 drops each of the essential oils of cypress and geranium. Or, make a mixture of these oils for traveling, and when needed, sprinkle a few drops on a handkerchief and inhale.

An essential oil taken from the cypress plant is suggested for menopause.

ACUPRESSURE

To ease problems associated with hormone changes, press your middle finger onto the point above the bridge of your nose halfway between your eyebrows. Apply gentle pressure for 2 minutes.

HOMEOPATHY

Hot flashes with a weepy mood, variable bleeding, and sleep disturbance may respond to

Lachesis is recommended for hot flashes

5

WHAT YOUR DOCTOR WOULD DO

Hormone replacement therapy (HRT) may be recommended by your doctor. This can be effective in dealing with any symptoms of menopause, and there is increasing evidence to suggest that it protects against osteoporosis and heart disease, too. The therapy consists of raising your estrogen toward its previous level. Because estrogen alone can have serious side effects, such as uterine or endometrial cancer, progestin is often included. This hormone, however, can have unpleasant side effects such as headaches, bloating, swollen breasts, and irregular bleeding. Your doctor will discuss the benefits and problems with you before you decide on the best approach. The hormones may be taken orally or as skin patches or gels.

Your doctor will suggest you stop smoking as it lowers the estrogen level. Increasing your calcium level may prevent osteoporosis. Foods high in calcium include dairy products, such as milk, cheese, and yogurt, sardines and salmon, calcium-fortified orange juice, broccoli, and beans. To absorb the calcium, your body needs vitamin D. Being outdoors in the sun allows your skin to make vitamin D but always use sunscreen to protect your skin during exposure to sun. Half an hour's exercise five times a week helps prevent osteoporosis and is also good for your heart.

CALL A DOCTOR IF

- You have vaginal bleeding after menopause
- Your symptoms cause you great discomfort
- You have a high risk of osteoporosis
- You have questions

Pulsatilla, or the more intense remedy *Lachesis*. To be sure, consult your prescriber on this important decision.

 HERBAL REMEDIES

A tea can be made using these herbs by steeping a teaspoon of the dried herb, or herbs, in a cup of hot water for 10 minutes and then straining it:
- You can combine chaste tree, wild yam, and

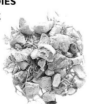
Wild yam is one of the herbs used to reduce hot flashes.

motherwort to make a tea for reducing the discomfort and frequency of hot flashes.
- To raise your estrogen levels, drink black cohosh tea.
- A nighttime drink to reduce sweating can be made by adding 3 drops of the essential oil of sage to hot water and honey.

The black cohosh plant improves estrogen levels.

5

DIAPER RASH & CRADLE CAP

SYMPTOMS

DIAPER RASH:
- The skin is red and dry around the buttocks, genitals, and thighs, and the baby may feel sore
- A strong smell of ammonia

CRADLE CAP:
- Yellowish or brownish greasy scales in patches or covering the whole head

CALL A DOCTOR IF

DIAPER RASH:
- The rash is severe or does not go away within a few days

A type of skin irritation in the area where a baby normally wears a diaper is known as diaper rash. Cradle cap is a type of dermatitis (see pp.66–67) in babies that usually appears in the first three months, but it can affect toddlers, too.

CAUSES
- Diaper rash is caused when a baby's skin is left in contact with a wet, soiled diaper, whether cloth or disposable, for too long. It can also occur if the baby is not dried properly after a bath or if there is an allergic reaction to soaps or lotions. Sometimes diaper rash is caused by yeast (thrush) or other infections.
- Cradle cap results from the accumulation of dead skin cells.

WHAT YOUR DOCTOR WOULD DO
As soon as you notice any redness on the baby's bottom, wash it with warm water and dry it completely. Gently apply a diaper rash cream, and avoid using rubber pants while the baby has the rash. For a severe case, the doctor may suggest over-the-counter yeast creams.

To treat cradle cap, rub baby oil or olive oil onto the baby's head. Leave the oil on for 24 hours, then gently comb through before washing the hair. Otherwise, buy special over-the-counter shampoos.

ALTERNATIVE TREATMENTS

HERBAL REMEDIES
- Comfrey or calendula ointments can soothe diaper rash and cradle cap.
- To relieve cradle cap, add a few drops of tea tree oil to a mild shampoo.

AROMATHERAPY
Mix 2 drops each of the essential oils of sandalwood, peppermint, and lavender oil in 4 tablespoons of a carrier oil, such as almond. Gently massage the mixture over the red area of a diaper rash.

Lavender essential oil can help relieve diaper rash.

PREVENTING DIAPER RASH

- Keep the baby's bottom as clean and dry as possible. Make sure it is washed properly and the diapers, either cloth or disposable, are changed regularly.
- Whenever possible, allow the baby to go without a diaper so that the skin is exposed to the air.
- To protect the skin from moisture, apply a barrier cream, such as one containing zinc and castor oil. Or use cornstarch instead of baby powder or talcum powder (both of which can inflame broken skin)—as long as the baby doesn't have a yeast infection, which thrives on cornstarch.

5

COLIC

Prolonged bouts of crying and irritability in a baby are known as colic. This occurs in about one out of five babies. Although it may cause frayed nerves in parents, colic has no lasting effects on the baby and usually disappears three months after it starts.

CAUSES
■ Sometimes colic is due to a harmless but unexplained spasm of the baby's intestines.

WHAT YOUR DOCTOR WOULD DO
If the baby is crying more than usual your doctor can help you rule out any serious problem.

You should check for reasons why the baby might be crying. For example, the air might be smoke-filled and irritating. Look for an open diaper pin or a diaper rash that might be making the baby uncomfortable, offer the baby the breast (or bottle) to make sure he or she isn't hungry or thirsty, or simply wants the comfort of sucking, or being close to you. Look for signs of illness.

Otherwise, try to soothe and distract the baby. Rhythmic activities such as rocking or a drive in the car can help, as can playing the static sound known as "white noise" from a radio that is set between stations. Wrapping the baby in a blanket or carrying him or her in a sling may provide a sense of comfort and security.

ALTERNATIVE TREATMENTS

AROMATHERAPY
To help relieve any discomfort associated with colic, gently massage the baby's stomach in a clockwise direction with 2 drops of the essential oil of fennel mixed into ½ teaspoon of a carrier oil such as almond or wheatgerm.

Gently massage the baby with fennel oil.

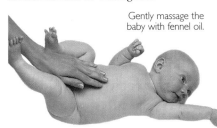

HERBAL REMEDIES
Chamomile or fennel tea may reduce gas in the baby's stomach. Steep a teaspoon of the herb in a cup of boiling water for 10 minutes and strain. Give the baby a teaspoon of the warm tea each hour but contact your doctor if the problem continues.

Dried chamomile can reduce gas.

5

ACUPRESSURE
To soothe crying, gently press the webbed area between the baby's thumb and index finger of each hand for 1 minute.

CHICKEN POX

Chicken pox is an infection that mainly affects children. Having it prevents you from getting it again.

CAUSES
- The herpes virus that causes shingles also causes chicken pox, which is very contagious. It spreads by sneezing, coughing, or contact with the skin rash.
- Children tolerate chicken pox very well. Previously unexposed teenagers and adults may get a more severe case of chicken pox.

WHAT YOUR DOCTOR WOULD DO
Your doctor may recommend acetaminophen or ibuprofen for the fever and antihistamines for the itching associated with the rash. Children are infectious and should be kept home from school until the fever is gone and the scabs have crusted over.

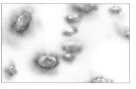

A chicken pox rash starts as spots on the chest and back. These turn to blisters, and the rash spreads to the face, arms, and legs. It disappears in 2 weeks.

ALTERNATIVE TREATMENTS

HERBAL REMEDIES
- An elderflower wash or a rosemary and calendula wash can soothe a chicken pox rash. Add 1 ounce (30 g) of elderflowers or 1 ounce (30 g) of each of the other 2 herbs to 1 quart (950 ml) of boiling water; simmer for 5 minutes.

Pot marigold is used to make a calendula wash.

Let the mixture cool and strain it. Soak a cloth in the liquid and apply it to the rash.

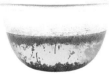

An infusion of elderflowers soothes a chicken pox rash.

ACUPRESSURE
For general pain relief, squeeze the web of the hand, between the thumb and forefinger, for 2 minutes. **Warning!** Do not do this if you are pregnant.

5

MEASLES, MUMPS, & RUBELLA

SYMPTOMS

MEASLES:
■ Fever, coughing, runny nose, and rash

MUMPS:
■ Swelling of the salivary glands, fever, and difficulty swallowing

RUBELLA:
■ Swollen glands; loss of appetite; possible rash

Warning!
Never give a child under 12 years of age aspirin—it can cause a serious illness called Reye's syndrome.

Measles, mumps, and rubella used to be common infections in childhood. Now that children are immunized, these illnesses have become uncommon.

CAUSES
■ Measles and mumps are caused by viruses and spread by coughing and sneezing.
■ Rubella (German Measles) is also also a virus. It can cause birth defects if a mother is infected during pregnancy.

WHAT YOUR DOCTOR WOULD DO
Always see the doctor for measles and mumps. He may advise painkillers for fever and discomfort and drinking lots of fluids. If you are pregnant and have been exposed to rubella, see your doctor right away.

In measles, red spots appear near the hairline and spread across the face and to the torso. They then spread to the legs and arms, and can merge to form irregular patches. The rash disappears after a week.

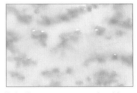

Rubella may cause a rash with tiny pink spots forming on the face and torso. After about 2 or 3 days, the rash on the face disappears, but a rash appears on the arms and legs, and lasts for up to 5 days.

ALTERNATIVE TREATMENTS

HERBAL REMEDIES
■ For a measles rash, mix a teaspoon of distilled witch hazel with ½ pint (250 ml) of water and sponge onto the rash.
■ A cooled infusion of lavender can also be soothing. Steep a teaspoon of the herb in a cup of boiling water for 10 minutes; let cool and strain.

Diluted witch hazel soothes a rash.

AT HOME CARE

MEASLES AND MUMPS:
■ Keep an infected child isolated while he or she is contagious: 8–12 days.
■ If the child's eyes are sensitive to light, keep the lights dim and restrict television viewing and reading.
■ To alleviate the itching of measles, apply a calamine lotion or a paste made with baking soda and water.

RUBELLA:
■ Keep the child home until a week after the rash disappears.
■ Sponge with cool water to reduce a fever and soothe the rash.

5

TEETHING PROBLEMS

SYMPTOMS

- Irritability and increased crying at night
- Chewing on fingers
- Drooling
- When a tooth is about to break through, inflamed swollen gum
- Difficulty in getting the baby to take milk, either from your breast or a bottle

CALL A DOCTOR IF

- Teeth do not appear by the time the child is 12 months old

When babies reach about six months old, teeth that have been developing beneath the gums since before birth begin to break through. In total, 20 teeth should appear, generally by the time the child is 3 years old. The speed at which the teeth emerge depends on hereditary factors.

CAUSES

- A tooth pushing through the gum can be irritating and may cause swelling where the tooth is about to emerge.
- The baby may refuse to take the bottle or breast because the mechanics of sucking bring blood to the swollen area, which increases the discomfort.

WHAT YOUR DOCTOR WOULD DO

If the pain appears to be severe, your doctor may recommend special painkillers. Otherwise, you can only try to make the baby more comfortable. A cloth with an ice cube in it can be gently stroked over the gums. Some babies enjoy chewing on a cooled teething ring. You can also gently rub the gum with your finger.

ALTERNATIVE TREATMENTS

HOMEOPATHY

Many people give only *Chamomilla* for teething irritability, but it is indicated in a specific circumstance—that of a child who is so irritable he or she cannot be soothed. Another remedy, *Calcarea carbonica*, may help a pale, chilly child with a chronically sweaty head who cannot seem to push the teeth through, getting stuck for weeks with each teething trial.

HERBAL REMEDIES

Syrup made from marsh mallow root may help reduce soreness in the gums.

Add 3 teaspoons of the syrup to the baby's food or drink every day.

AROMATHERAPY

To relax the baby, add 2 drops of the essential oils of chamomile or lavender to a vaporizer in the baby's room.

ACUPRESSURE

To help reduce the baby's pain, using your thumb and index finger, gently massage the web of skin between the baby's thumb and index finger. Repeat on the other hand.

5

Emotional Conditions

Alternative Health

EMOTIONAL CONDITIONS

With the hectic pace of life today, many people struggle to balance their family life with demanding hours at work. While some stress is beneficial and can even improve performance, prolonged periods of pressure can affect our health, causing conditions such as insomnia and depression. Other events in our lives, such as a death in the family or divorce, can also cause emotional upsets.

Our mental health can also suffer from ailments such as anxiety, which can be triggered by extreme stress or by hereditary conditions. Even a lack of light during short winter days can lead to a form of depression known as seasonal affective disorder. You should know that these conditions are not unusual, and they are all treatable.

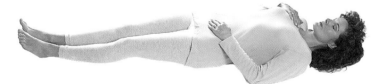

STRESS

- Headaches
- Fatigue
- Dry mouth
- Heart palpitation
- Insomnia
- Irritability
- Tearfulness
- Muscle aches
- Diarrhea or constipation
- Skin rashes
- More likely to catch a cold or the flu
- Change in appetite, eating either more or less than normal
- More likely to worry about trivial matters
- Less interest in sex

Humans once had to deal with life or death situations on a daily basis when they had to protect themselves from predators. Our bodies coped with these situations using a "flight or fight" response, in which the heart beats faster, the pupils in the eyes expand, and the muscles tense to help the body react quickly. Nowadays, the flight or fight response may become activated simply by the strains of everyday living. A feeling of being overstressed occurs when we have difficulty handling these demands.

CAUSES

- An illness or death in the family can cause symptoms of stress.
- The breakdown of a marriage is stressful, not only in the adults, but also in any children involved.
- The birth of a child is often stressful.
- Moving to a new house can be very stressful.
- Pressure at work causes stress problems.
- Stress symptoms are often caused by financial difficulties.
- Positive experiences, such as getting married, buying a house or a job promotion can be stressful.
- Some individuals become overstressed simply by making everyday decisions, such as what to cook for supper, what to wear to a special event, or where to go on vacation. ▶

ALTERNATIVE TREATMENTS

HERBAL REMEDIES
Chamomile or passion-flower tea can soothe stress. Steep a teaspoon of the dried herb in a cup of boiling water for 10 minutes, then strain.

Passionflower can be soothing when taken as a tea.

AROMATHERAPY
Put 5 or 6 drops of lavender essential oil into a hot bath and relax. Or, add 1 or 2 drops of the oil to a handkerchief and inhale the scent.

REFLEXOLOGY
Working on the reflexology point for the adrenal glands can help reduce stress, while the point for the solar plexus can help you relax. Apply pressure to these points for 1 minute each on both feet.

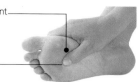

Reflexology point for the adrenal glands

Reflexology point for the solar plexus

6

WHAT YOUR DOCTOR WOULD DO

You may initially visit your doctor for one of the symptoms rather than the stress itself, but she may be able to diagnose stress as the problem by recognizing the physical and psychological symptoms. Once the problem is identified, your doctor may suggest ways of tackling the aspects of your lifestyle that are causing the problem. In severe cases, such as when coming to terms with the death of a loved one, an anti-anxiety drug may be recommended for short-term relief.

To help you cope with stress your doctor may suggest the following:

■ Work out what is making you stressed. If you feel that you have too much to do, make a list of your tasks for the day, putting essential ones at the top. Learn to delegate some of the tasks and move less important ones to later in the week.

■ Exercise makes the body release chemicals that act as natural antidepressants. Take part in an activity you enjoy, perhaps with a friend.

■ Don't rely on alcohol and tobacco. They only make you feel worse in the long run. Try to eat a healthy diet and avoid turning to junk food.

■ Take time off. Make sure you have at least an hour a day just for yourself. Go for a walk, soak in the bathtub, or unplug the telephone and read.

CALL A DOCTOR IF

■ You experience prolonged stress symptoms, as these can increase your susceptibility to certain serious disorders

VISUALIZATION

A progressive muscle relaxation technique can reduce stress. Each group of muscles is tensed and then relaxed from head to toe. It takes about 15 minutes and can be practiced a few times a week while lying in a quiet room.

Take deep, slow breaths so that your stomach rises but not your chest. Tense each of the muscle groups for a count of 5, then relax them. Start with your eyebrows and forehead. For your jaw and face, open your mouth as wide as you can; then tense your neck and shoulder muscles. Lift your arms and tense them; then tense your rib and stomach muscles. One at a time, raise your legs and tense them and your feet. Lie still for a few minutes, imagining yourself in a special place, such as on a beach or in a forest.

You can listen to quiet music while practicing the technique.

6

INSOMNIA

Insomnia is the inability to sleep through the night and is an extremely common complaint. There are three main types:
- Transient insomnia: a temporary disruption of sleeping patterns that lasts for only a few nights.
- Short-term insomnia: a temporary difficulty in sleeping that lasts for a few weeks.
- Chronic insomnia: being deprived of sleep over a long period of time; this can have certain serious effects on a person's health.

Causes
- Traveling to a new place in a different time zone can cause transient insomnia. This type of insomnia can also be caused when your working hours change, particularly if you do shift work.
- Environmental factors can cause insomnia, including noise, lights, sunshine, or a stuffy room.
- Inconsistent sleeping habits may cause insomnia, for example, if you nap during the day or go to bed at a different hour each night.
- Insomnia is often caused by alcohol, caffeine, and certain over-the-counter and prescription medicines.
- Stress and other psychological factors frequently cause insomnia.
- Certain disorders, such as heartburn, chronic pain, and diabetes, sometimes cause insomnia. ▶

ALTERNATIVE TREATMENTS

HOMEOPATHY

Insomnia can have many causes. Depending on the individual circumstance, specific homeopathy remedies may be very helpful.
- If you cannot get to sleep from racing thoughts, try *Nux vomica* in a 12 or 30c potency. Repeat after an hour if you are still awake
- If one specific phrase or musical tune is interfering with sleep, try first *Pulsatilla*, as above.

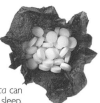

Nux vomica can help improve sleep.

HERBAL REMEDIES

- For a good night's sleep, steep 2 teaspoons of dried, chopped valerian root in a cup of boiling water and let stand for 8 hours. Strain, sweeten and drink before going to bed.
Warning! Valerian may impair your ability to drive or operate machinery.

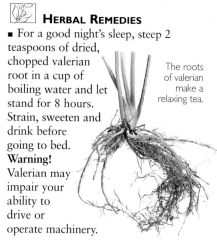

The roots of valerian make a relaxing tea.

6

WHAT YOUR DOCTOR WOULD DO

Transient insomnia should stop once your body has had a chance to become used to any new routine; it normally does not require treatment.

For short-term and chronic insomnia, the doctor will treat the underlying problem causing your sleeplessness. She'll examine you to look for a physical cause for the condition; for example, an overactive thyroid gland. If there isn't a physical cause, she'll ask you about any emotional upsets that may be stopping you from sleeping; a therapist may be recommended. Sleeping tablets may be prescribed for the short term. Suggestions for helping you sleep may include:

- Go to bed only when you are tired. If you can't sleep, get up. Don't lie in bed tossing and turning.
- Make sure your bed is comfortable and that the room is warm or cool enough.
- Don't go to bed with a full or empty stomach.
- Avoid drinking caffeine in the evenings.
- Don't turn to alcohol; it can disturb your sleep and leave you feeling more tired in the long run.
- If you want a late night snack, eat a banana. This is a good source of a chemical—tryptophan—that can relax and calm you.

CALL A DOCTOR IF

- You have trouble sleeping for more than a month
- You are taking a prescribed medicine to help you sleep but it is no longer effective

- A tea made with chamomile or lime blossoms can help calm you. Add a teaspoon of the herb to a cup of boiling water and steep for 10 minutes before straining it. You should drink a cup before going to bed.

AROMATHERAPY

The essential oils of chamomile, neroli, lavender, and rose all have properties to help you relax. Before going to bed, add several drops of one of the oils to a warm bath. Or sprinkle a few drops on a handkerchief and inhale the scent.

ACUPRESSURE

To help reduce anxiety and promote sleep, you can apply pressure with your index fingers to the points 2 fingers' width behind each ear and press for 1 minute.

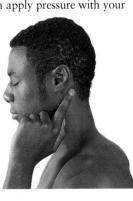

Acupressure points behind the ears reduce anxiety.

6

DEPRESSION

SYMPTOMS

- Feelings of disliking or hating yourself
- Lack of interest or enjoyment of life
- Feeling guilty and blaming yourself for things that go wrong
- Extreme tiredness and lack of energy
- Insomnia or sleeping too much
- Reduced or increased appetite
- Lowered sex drive
- Thoughts of suicide
- Sluggish movements or speech

Everyone has days when they feel low or sad, due usually to some event or situation in their lives. In true depression, the depressed person not only feels low, but also has difficulty in coping with normal activities. A common illness that affects up to 50 percent of women and 25 percent of men at some time in their lives, depression has several categories:
- A depressive reaction is a type of minor, temporary depression that is a response to a specific life situation. It goes away in two weeks to six months.
- Dysthymia is also a type of minor, temporary depression but lasts for up to two years.
- Major depression is a serious condition that can lead to thoughts of suicide. It appears suddenly without a trigger and goes away just as suddenly, perhaps in six months to a year. It tends to be cyclical so it may return.

CAUSES

- A depressive reaction is usually caused by a major life event, such as death or a marriage breakdown; a reaction to a medication; hormonal changes, such as before menstruation or after childbirth; and illnesses such as a viral infection or chronic pain or fatigue.
- Dysthymia and major depression may be caused by an imbalance of certain brain chemicals called neurotransmitters. ▶

ALTERNATIVE TREATMENTS

ACUPRESSURE

To help alleviate depression, use your index finger to press gently in the groove above the upper lip and below the nose for 1 minute.

Acupressure point above the lip reduces depression.

HERBAL REMEDIES

- Borage, St John's wort or vervain tea may help raise your spirits.
- St John's wort in capsule form can also help. Take 300 mg 2–3 times daily
- Rosemary tea can also help make you feel less depressed.

Steep a teaspoon of dried, crushed rosemary leaves in a cup of boiling water for 10 minutes. Strain before drinking the tea.

Borage can help reduce depression.

WHAT YOUR DOCTOR WOULD DO

Your doctor may prescribe antidepressant drugs. These have come a long way in recent years and some are often no longer addictive; indeed many people find drugs can be very helpful in getting them through a period of depression. Your doctor will also be able to put you in touch with a counsellor or therapist if you need to talk through your worries. Your doctor may also suggest you take some of the following measures to help you get through the episode:

- Try to involve your partner instead of trying to manage your depression on your own. Tell your partner how you are feeling. It may also help to talk to your friends.
- Get some brisk exercise for half an hour 5 times a week. Although it may be the last thing you feel like doing, physical activity releases endorphins—natural antidepressant chemicals—in the body.
- Don't turn to alcohol, cigarettes or junk food—they can make you feel worse.
- If you can, take a short break away.
- Remember what you used to do to give you pleasure and try to include these activities in your day to day life.

CALL A DOCTOR IF

- You or a member of your family has thoughts of suicide
- You or a member of your family has had symptoms for more than a few weeks

REFLEXOLOGY

Several reflexology points help combat depression. Apply pressure to each one for 1 minute. Repeat on the other foot.

- Stimulate the 3 points for the head, which are located on the bottom of the big toe: at the base, the outside edge and the top of the toe.

- To aid relaxation, apply pressure to the solar plexus point, which is to the side of the ball of the foot.
- To reduce stress, press on the point for the adrenal glands at the ball of the foot, near the solar plexus reflex.

AROMATHERAPY

Essential oils of jasmine, bergamot, lavender, clary sage, rose, and chamomile can be uplifting. Add a few drops of one of the oils to your bath, or put the oil into a bowl of hot water to scent a room. Alternatively, put a few drops on a handkerchief and inhale the scent.

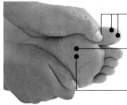

Reflexology points for the head

Reflexology point for the adrenal glands

Reflexology point for the solar plexus

6

ANXIETY

SYMPTOMS

- Sweating
- Unreasonable sense of danger or worry
- Dry mouth
- Heart palpitation
- Chest pains
- Inability to concentrate
- Tense muscles
- Hyperventilation

CALL A DOCTOR IF

- You seem to over-react to a situation
- Anxiety gets in the way of your normal activities
- You feel anxious for several weeks
- You suddenly have severe symptoms

Most people have feelings of anxiety during times of danger or stress. But experiencing disproportionate anxiety or anxious feelings when there is no clear cause is distressing and debilitating. Anxiety comes in many forms: a panic attack is a sudden and extreme fear for no obvious reason; phobias are fears of common items, including spiders, schools, dentists, water, heights and, enclosed spaces; and obsessive-compulsive disorders occur when anxiety and other emotions cause unnecessarily repeated actions, such as washing the hands repeatedly.

CAUSES
- Stress from an accident, illness, death in the family, or financial problems often cause anxiety.
- An unhappy or frightening event that occurred during childhood, even though it is not consciously remembered, can lead to anxiety in adulthood.
- Anxiety may be an inherited trait.

WHAT YOUR DOCTOR WOULD DO
The doctor will examine you to rule out any physical causes, such as thyroid or heart problems. If nothing is found, you may be advised to see a therapist to find out what is making you feel anxious. You may be prescribed anti-anxiety drugs, but these can be addictive so they are only recommended in the short term.

ALTERNATIVE TREATMENTS

AROMATHERAPY
Rub a few drops of the essential oils of jasmine, lavender, or chamomile into the temples, or add them to a tissue and inhale.

Inhale lavender oil to reduce anxiety

HERBAL REMEDIES
Steep a teaspoon of dried lemon balm, dried chamomile, or linden flowers in a cup of boiling water for 10 minutes and strain.

VISUALIZATION
Lying down, place one hand on your abdomen and the other on your chest. Breathe in so that you feel your abdomen rise substantially, while your chest hardly moves. Take 8 breaths a minute, then slow the rhythm. Once you have established a steady rhythm, imagine yourself in a quiet place, such as on a deserted beach or sunny hillside.

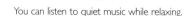

You can listen to quiet music while relaxing.

6

PANIC ATTACKS

SYMPTOMS

- Rapid and shallow breathing, or a feeling that you cannot breathe
- Heart palpitation
- Sweating and shaking
- Feeling dizzy or faint
- Numbness or tingling in the hands or feet
- Feeling nauseous
- Feelings of unreality and terror

CALL A DOCTOR IF

- You believe that you might have a panic disorder
- You think you might be having a heart attack—the symptoms can be similar

A panic attack is an unconsciously exaggerated response to fear, stress, or excitement. Once such an attack has been experienced, people often become panicky at the thought of it happening again, so another panic attack can be triggered simply by the fear of having one.

CAUSES

- Panic attacks may be caused by a chemical imbalance in your system.
- Extreme stress—which may occur when a family member is ill or dies, or with a marriage breakdown—may trigger panic attacks.
- Some medical problems can cause attacks, as can certain medicines.

WHAT YOUR DOCTOR WOULD DO

As with anxiety, there can be physical causes of panic attacks, so your doctor will rule those out first. If there is no physical cause, you will be reassured that the feelings, however dramatic and unpleasant, cannot harm you and will pass eventually. You may be advised to you see a therapist who specializes in panic disorders.

ALTERNATIVE TREATMENTS

HERBAL REMEDIES

Infusions made from skullcap, vervain, or lemon balm can help soothe the symptoms of a panic attack. To make an infusion, steep 1 teaspoon of the dried herb in a cup of boiling water for 10 minutes and strain.

AROMATHERAPY

The lavender essential oil is effective in relieving anxiety and stress. It is a good idea to carry a bottle with you; when needed, place a few drops of the oil either on a tissue or handkerchief and inhale the scent.

ACUPRESSURE

To relieve a panic attack, with your hand held palm upward, press your thumb firmly into your wrist on the same side as your little finger, about 1 finger's width into your arm. Massage the area in small circles for 3 minutes, then repeat on the other arm.

Acupressure point near the wrist can reduce anxious feelings.

6

SEASONAL AFFECTIVE DISORDER

SYMPTOMS

- Depression; lack of enjoyment in life
- Lethargy and extreme tiredness
- Oversleeping and overeating
- Cravings for carbohydrates
- Anxiety and irritability
- Loss of sex drive

CALL A DOCTOR IF

- You or a member of your family experience any of these symptoms during the winter months

Also known as SAD, seasonal affective disorder is a form of depression that affects people during the dark winter months—it is also known as the "winter blues."

CAUSES

- What causes SAD is still a mystery but low levels of serotonin, a chemical in the brain, may be responsible. The levels are at their lowest in winter when there is the least amount of outdoor light.
- Stress and lack of exercise make the condition worse.

WHAT YOUR DOCTOR WOULD DO

Many people seem to benefit from light therapy during the winter months. A special box that emits a light about 20 times brighter than normal indoor light is used by simply sitting in front of it for a number of hours each day. (Don't confuse this with a sunbed, which emits ultraviolet light and won't work, as well as being bad for the skin.) In some cases the doctor may prescribe antidepressants.

ALTERNATIVE TREATMENTS

AROMATHERAPY

To relieve feelings of sadness, add 6 to 8 drops of the essential oils of clary sage, Roman chamomile, or rose to a warm bath or place them in a bowl of hot water to scent a room. Or, carry a bottle with you; when needed, put a drop on a handkerchief and inhale the scent.

HOMEOPATHY

Treatments depend on the individual, so a consultation with a professional is advised.

WINTERTIME SELF-HELP

- Try to spend some time outside in the daylight each day.
- Go outside in the middle of the day for a 30-minute walk, even if it is a cloudy day.
- Try to work in front of a window. If necessary, trim any tree branches and shrubs near the window to allow as much light in as possible.
- Consider taking a vacation during winter in a place with longer days and brighter sun.

6

ALTERNATIVE HEALTH

There are many treatments in conventional medicine that are directly related to the *principles of some alternative health therapies. For example, like herbal remedies, aspirin was originally derived from a plant, and homeopathy works on the same principles as vaccines.*

Alternative therapies, some of which have been around for thousands of years, are often used to complement conventional medicine. These include herbal remedies and acupressure. Others, such as aromatherapy and reflexology, are relatively new, but their proponents are firm believers in the results.

If you become ill, it is always best to see your doctor first, but alternative therapies to 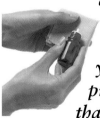 *alleviate the symptoms can be used alongside your doctor's recommendations—as long as you remember to inform your practitioner about any remedies that you may be taking.*

HOMEOPATHY

THE MAKING OF A REMEDY

A Homeopathic remedy is made by pulverizing a substance —such as a plant or mineral—in a suitable solvent, for example grain alcohol. The extract is diluted by a fixed amount, shaken to impart energy to the mixture, and diluted again. This is repeated many times, and the number and magnitude of the dilutions determine the number and letter of the potency. "30c" represents 30 dilutions of 1/100, with shaking between each one. The final solution is soaked into identical "blank" sugar pellets to make the actual remedy as sold to the consumer.

TAKING A REMEDY

Remedies are sensitive. Handle the pellets as little as possible—tap 2 or 3 into the lid of the bottle and without touching the inside of the lid, toss them into the mouth. Allow the pellets to dissolve under the tongue. For best results, do not eat, drink, or brush your teeth for 15 minutes before or after taking your dose.

HOW IT WORKS

Homeopathy is a system of medicine that was developed in the 1790s by the German physician Samuel Hahnemann. The doctor noticed that an herbal remedy for malaria (the herb used was later found to contain quinine—the first medicine used to treat malaria) produced the same symptoms in a healthy person. He deduced that the symptoms were nature's way of fighting the disease—a theory expressed by the Greek physician Hippocrates 2,300 years earlier. So Homeopathy is based on the idea of curing "like with like." In other words, elements that can cause the symptoms of a particular illness can, in the right doses, be used to cure it. Vaccines work on this principle: they are made from dead or live viruses and, when injected, provide immunity to the disease itself.

Science is just beginning to theorize about how such minute quantities of substances can have an effect on people (and animals), but 200 years of Homeopathic practitioners and millions of people worldwide can attest from personal experience to the efficacy of this unique healing system.

CONSTITUTIONAL VS SYMPTOMATIC TREATMENT

Homeopathy goes far beyond the simple symptom relief in this book. Homeopaths come to understand you as a whole person, not just a collection of symptoms. By treating the roots of your illness, a profound and lasting transformation is allowed to take place in your body and mind, removing the need for your person to react in the way that is causing suffering. "Constitutional" treatment is best for chronic serious illness. The remedies given in this book are suited for the treatment of common, acute ailments and may serve as an introduction to the larger body of Homeopathic medicine.

ANTIDOTING AND CONCURRENT TREATMENT

Always inform your Homeopath of any conventional or herbal medicines you are taking, and seek advice before attempting any self-prescribing. Avoid strongly aromatic scents, including menthol, strong mint, eucalyptus, and tea tree oil while under Homeopathic care.

HOMEOPATHY FIRST AID KIT

You can take the appropriate remedy every 2 hours for up to 6 doses. For information on doses and taking a remedy, see the boxes on the opposite page.

SOURCE	USED FOR
Apis 30c from honeybees	Allergic reactions in the eyes, throat, and mouth; sore throats; hives; cystitis; and insect stings. **Warning!** Do not use if pregnant.
Arnica 6c or 30c from *Arnica montana* (the leopard's bane flower)	Burns; stings; bruising; black eyes; nose bleeds; cuts and abrasions; cramps; sprains and strained muscles; arthritis; shock after injury; eczema; and whooping cough.
Bryonia 30c from the root of *Bryonia alba* (common bryony, wild hops)	Headaches; colds and the flu; nausea; heat exhaustion; painful breasts; and arthritis.
Cantharis 6c or 30c from a secretion made by the beetle called Spanish fly	Burns and scalds; blisters; burning or stinging sensations; and cystitis.
Euphrasia 6c from *Euphrasia officinalis* (the herb eyebright)	Conjunctivitis; eyestrain or eye injuries; and constipation.
Hypericum 30c from *Hypericum* (the herb St John's wort)	Cuts and abrasions; discomfort after dental treatment; head wounds; wounds with shooting pains; injuries that affect the nerves; depression; indigestion; nausea; and diarrhea.
Nux vomica 6c from *Strychnos nux vomica* (poison nut tree)	Colds and the flu; heavy periods; morning sickness; labor pains; frequent urination in pregnancy; cystitis; motion sickness; digestive problems; hangovers; and insomnia.
Silicea 6c from the mineral silica, found in many rocks	Recurring colds and infections; acne; and migraines.
Tabacum 6c from *Nicotiana tabacum* (tobacco plant)	Nausea and vomiting; motion sickness; faintness and dizziness; and anxiety.
Urtica 6c from *Urtica urens* (dwarf stinging nettle plant)	Burns and scalds; hives and other skin allergies; and cystitis.

6

HERBAL REMEDIES

MAKING AN INFUSION

To make an herbal infusion, or tea, put 1 or 2 teaspoons of the dried herb into a cup. Fill the cup with boiling water and steep, or let stand, for 10 minutes. Strain the tea, then add honey or sugar to mask any bitter or unpleasant taste.

If using fresh herbs, use 2 to 4 teaspoons. To make larger quantities, use ½ to 1 ounce (15–30 g) of dried herb (double the amount of fresh herb) for every 2 cups (500 ml) of water. Teas lose their medicinal qualities when exposed to air for a few hours. Store in a tightly sealed jar in the refrigerator for up to 3 days and warm gently when needed.

Warning!
Pregnant and breastfeeding women should always consult a qualified herbal practitioner before taking any remedy. There are some herbs which should **never** be taken in pregnancy, or given to an infant.

HOW THEY WORK

A variety of plant parts—flowers, fruit, leaves, roots, stems, bark, and seeds—are used to prepare herbal medicines. These contain ingredients that can help heal, cure, or relieve symptoms. Herbal medicine is one of the oldest forms of medicine. The slaves who built the pyramids in Egypt thousands of years ago ate garlic every day to avoid catching infections. Today, about one quarter of conventional medicines include some type of active ingredient derived from plants. Herbal remedies often taken longer to work than conventional medicine, partly because they are used in less concentrated forms.

WHAT TO EXPECT FROM A PRACTITIONER

Instead of treating a symptom directly, herbalists try to restore what they call the vital force—the body's own healing ability. A practitioner will ask about your lifestyle, diet, and emotional state before choosing a remedy, and will also want to know about your medical history and any conventional medicines that you may be taking. The remedy will then be prescribed in the lowest dose that will work.

Herbal remedies can be found in health food stores or specialty suppliers and are sold as tea bags; pills, capsules, and powders; extracts, and tinctures —types of concentrated liquids; and lotions, creams, and ointments. Herbs are also available for making your own teas (or infusions), compresses, poultices, tinctures, and ointments at home. Herbs are best absorbed on an empty stomach. If an herb makes you feel ill, take it with food. If headaches, diarrhea, or nausea consistently occur within 2 hours, tell your herbalist, who will change the remedy.

CAN I TREAT MYSELF?

The most effective treatments for serious or chronic conditions are best prescribed by a qualified practitioner of herbal medicine. In general, herbal remedies should be discussed with a practitioner because some herbs can be toxic if taken in the wrong concentrations. You can buy some of your own remedies, however, for certain common minor illnesses but consult your doctor if the symptoms persist or worsen, or if new ones appear, or if you are taking any conventional medicine.

COMMON HERBAL REMEDIES

These herbs can easily be found in health food stores or at specialist suppliers, and the remedies can be used at home safely.

HERB	USES
Burdock *Arctium lappa*	As a compress: use on cuts and abrasions. Soak a cloth in burdock tea before applying to the wound. As a decoction: take for fungal and bacterial infections; eczema and psoriasis; cystitis; and arthritis. Boil 1 teaspoon of the chopped root in 3 cups water for 30 minutes.
Calendula *Calendula officinalis*	As an infusion (see opposite): take 2 to 4 times daily for indigestion and period problems. Do not use if pregnant. As a lotion or ointment: rub on cuts and abrasions; measles and chicken pox rashes; and diaper rash and athlete's foot. .
German chamomile *Chamomilla recutita* (also known as *Matricaria recutita*)	As an infusion of the flowers (see opposite): take 3 to 4 times daily for indigestion; menstrual cramps and colic; and just before bedtime for insomnia. As a compress: use for swelling, painful joints; inflamed skin and sunburn; cuts and abrasions; hemorrhoids; and sore eyes. Soak the cloth in a strained infusion at room temperature diluted with an equal part of water.
Comfrey *Symphytum officinale*	As a poultice: for cuts; insect bites; bruises; and inflamed skin. Shake the powder over the affected area and cover with a clean bandage. **Warning!** Never take comfrey internally.
Eyebright *Euphrasia officinalis*	As an infusion (see opposite): drink 3 cups daily for stuffy noses; coughs from colds; sinusitis; and allergies. As a compress: apply to eyes irritated by hay fever or other allergies; colds; and conjunctivitis. Dip a clean cloth in a strained infusion at room temperature; apply for 15 minutes.
Hyssop *Hyssopus officinalis*	As an infusion (see opposite): drink 3 times a day for colds, coughs, and bronchitis; indigestion and gas; and anxiety. As a compress (soak a clean cloth in 2 batches of the infusion): use for cold sores; burns; cuts; and other skin irritations.
Lavender *Lavandula officinalis*	As an infusion (see opposite): drink 3 times a day for insomnia or depression; headache; stress; indigestion; nausea; and gas.
Stinging nettle *Urtica dioica*	As an infusion (see opposite): drink 2 times a day for hay fever; eczema; yeast infections; premenstrual syndrome; heavy periods; diarrhea; cystitis; hemorrhoids; arthritis; and gout.

6

AROMATHERAPY

MASSAGE

Add a few drops of an essential oil to 2 ounces (60 ml) of a carrier oil, such as apricot kernel or almond. This will make enough for a back massage. You can massage the parts of your body that you can reach yourself by rubbing the oil into your skin, but you'll need someone else to give you a full body massage.

OTHER WAYS TO USE THE OILS

■ In the bath: add about 5 drops of the essential oil to warm bath water, stir, settle in, and relax.
■ As a compress: add 4–5 drops to a bowl of water. Soak a clean cloth in it, picking up as much of the oil as you can; wring it out and apply to the affected area. Use hot water for muscle pain and arthritis, and cold water for headaches, sprains, and swellings.
■ As an inhalation: put 3–4 drops in a bowl of hot water. Bend your head over the bowl. Cover up with a towel to catch the steam. Or put a few drops on a clean handkerchief and inhale the aroma.

HOW IT WORKS

The oil extracted from certain plants is believed to have the ability to relax people and to relieve the symptoms of certain disorders. This practice of using essential oils has been a part of human history for thousands of years. In fact, ancient Chinese documents describe the importance that aromas play in promoting both physical health and spirituality.

The fragrance of the essential oils affects the part of the brain that controls memory, emotion, and hormone levels. Some oils are also absorbed through the skin and carried throughout the body by the bloodstream and lymph. In particular, the oils can benefit muscular pains; digestive disorders; symptoms of menstruation and menopause; stress-related problems; depression; and insomnia.

WHAT TO EXPECT FROM A PRACTITIONER

The practitioner will usually begin the first visit by asking you a series of questions about yourself and your problem. This information helps her to find out about your general health and lifestyle, including your diet, exercise, posture, and sleeping habits. A selection of essential oils will be chosen and blended together. The mixture will be given to you to take home. The practitioner may also give you a massage treatment during the visit.

CAN I TREAT MYSELF?

You can use the essential oils at home for certain common disorders and they can be used in combinations. You should always buy high-quality oils from a specialist supplier to make sure you get pure essential oils. Unless you are using tree tea oil, don't apply the oil directly to your skin—the oils are concentrated and can cause irritation. There are many ways to use the oils, including massage, in a bath, inhalation, and as a compress (see left). Sometimes essential oils may be recommended as a gargle, but unless you are following instructions from a qualified practitioner, this should not be practiced because it can be dangerous.
Warning! If you are pregnant, always consult a qualified practitioner first—there are a number of oils that pregnant women should avoid.

COMMON ESSENTIAL OILS

Below are some suggestions for using common essential oils. Although specific methods of using an oil for certain conditions are given below, others may also be appropriate. For various ways of using the oils, see the boxes on the opposite page. **Caution!** Some aromatic oils, such as tea tree, neutralize homeopathic remedies.

ESSENTIAL OILS	USES
Chamomile *Chamomilla recutita* and *Chamomilla nobile* (also known as *Matricaria recutita* and *Matricaria nobile*)	**As a massage:** for menstrual cramps and heavy periods; muscle pain and arthritic pain; insomnia, anxiety, and stress; and indigestion and gas. **In a bath:** for stress, anxiety and insomnia. **With a few drops on a cotton ball or swab:** dab on acne, eczema, cuts, and abrasions.
Eucalyptus *Eucalyptus globulus*	**In an inhalation:** for coughs, colds, the flu, sinusitis, and bronchitis. **As a massage:** good for muscle aches and fibrositis. **On a compress:** soothes insect bites and rashes from chicken pox or shingles. **With a few drops on a cotton ball or swab:** dab on cuts, abrasions, bruises, and burns.
Lavender *Lavandula angustifolia*	**As a massage:** for muscle aches; colic; stomach ache, nausea, indigestion, and gas; and stress, depression, and insomnia. **In a bath:** for stress, depression and insomnia. **In an inhalation:** for congestion, colds, the flu, rhinitis, and bronchitis. **On a compress:** for burns, bruises, acne, hives, and insect bites.
Rosemary *Romarinus officinalis*	**As a massage:** for muscle aches and strains; menstrual cramps; and fluid retention. **In an inhalation:** for colds, coughs, congestion, and headaches. **On a compress:** for muscle aches; sprains; headaches; indigestion; and gas. **In a bath:** for menstrual cramps and fluid retention.
Tea tree *Melaleuca alternifolia*	**Applied directly to the skin:** for cuts, insect stings, cold sores, canker sores, and warts. **In an inhalation:** for colds, the flu, and sinusitis. **On a compress:** for blisters; rashes from chicken pox and shingles, and other rashes.

6

ACUPRESSURE

HOW IT WORKS

One of a number of treatments used in traditional Chinese medicine, acupressure is based on applying pressure to precise points on the body to strengthen, calm or unblock the flow of "chi," or vital energy. These points are located on meridians—pathways in the body, which correspond with blood vessels or nerves. There are two sets of 12 meridians that run along each side of the body and have the same points. Two additional meridians run down the center of the body. By applying pressure to a point, a particular symptom can be relieved; pressing several points in a certain order can improve the well-being of the body as a whole. Research has shown that acupressure relieves nausea and pain.

Each point is linked to an organ that affects bodily functions. The points are named and numbered, according to which meridians they are on. They may be used to treat ailments other than those indicated.

Governing Vessel 24.5, to relieve hay fever

Stomach 3, to relieve sinus headaches

Large Intestine 11, for inflammation, hormone imbalance, and emotional upset of acne; to relieve constipation and fever

Lung 5, to reduce coughing bouts

Stomach 25, to reduce pain in irritable bowel syndrome

Conception Vessel 6, to reduce abdominal pains from constipation

Conception Vessel 4, to correct irregular periods

Large Intestine 4, to reduce skin irritation, muscle aches, constipation, hay fever, and headaches

Liver 8, to reduce the effects of depression

Spleen 10, to stimulate the immune system

Stomach 36, to relieve abdominal pain, nausea, and indigestion and to boost immunity stystem

Spleen 6, to reduce water retention and colic

Liver 3, to decrease headaches and menstrual cramps

Liver 4, to promote health of female reproductive organs

WHAT TO EXPECT FROM A PRACTITIONER

The therapist will ask a series of questions to find out about your general health, diet, and lifestyle. You'll then be asked to sit or lie down on a table or mattress so that the practitioner can proceed with the therapy. There are several techniques, and they differ in the combination of points used and the way the pressure is applied. Massage is typically used during the procedure.

CAN I TREAT MYSELF?

Many of the points for common symptoms can be used at home. Be careful that you don't overstimulate the point because this may cause a worsening of the symptoms for a short period.

> **Warning!**
> Never apply pressure to the abdomen or on Spleen 6 or Large Intestine 4 if you are pregnant.
>
> Do not apply pressure where there is an open wound, infected or inflamed skin, tumor, varicose vein, a possible broken bone, or near a recent surgical scar.

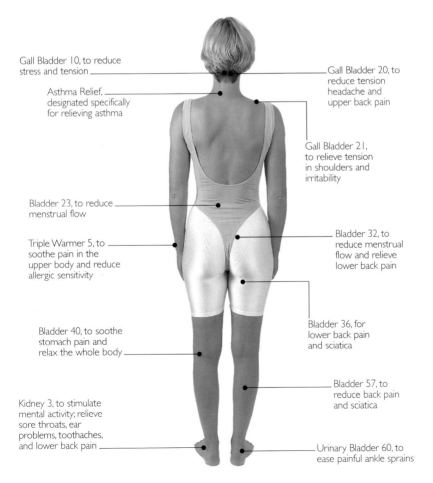

Gall Bladder 10, to reduce stress and tension

Asthma Relief, designated specifically for relieving asthma

Gall Bladder 20, to reduce tension headache and upper back pain

Gall Bladder 21, to relieve tension in shoulders and irritability

Bladder 23, to reduce menstrual flow

Bladder 32, to reduce menstrual flow and relieve lower back pain

Triple Warmer 5, to soothe pain in the upper body and reduce allergic sensitivity

Bladder 36, for lower back pain and sciatica

Bladder 40, to soothe stomach pain and relax the whole body

Bladder 57, to reduce back pain and sciatica

Kidney 3, to stimulate mental activity; relieve sore throats, ear problems, toothaches, and lower back pain

Urinary Bladder 60, to ease painful ankle sprains

6

REFLEXOLOGY

Always use your thumb to put pressure on a reflex point. Bend the thumb first and keep it bent. Using the tip of your thumb—not the nail—press on the point for about a minute, then gently release the pressure without unbending your thumb. If you are doing a series of points, move onto the next point, keeping your thumb bent and as close to the foot as possible.

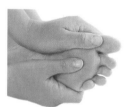

Support the foot with one hand while the other hand is massaging and applying the pressure. Always hold the foot firmly but comfortably.

Warning!
Never have reflexology on your feet if you suffer from thrombosis.

See a practitioner if you have diabetes; don't try reflexology techniques on your feet on your own.

HOW IT WORKS
This type of foot massage, which concentrates on specific areas of the feet to treat certain medical conditions, is known as reflexology, or zone therapy. Based on similar theories found in traditional Chinese treatments, reflexology works on the principle that energy from the entire body flows to the feet. If this energy becomes blocked, it can have an effect on the health of the body.

Although similar foot therapies have been used by other cultures in the past, reflexology is basically a modern treatment—it was developed in the early 20th century by an American physician, Dr. William Fitzgerald. He created maps of the feet, showing the areas that correspond with parts of the body. For example, sections of the big toe represent the head and brain. Following Fitzgerald's theory, it is possible to reduce pain from a headache by applying reflexology techniques to the big toe. Reflexology points are also found on the hands, but these are not considered as effective as those on the feet.

WHAT TO EXPECT FROM A PRACTITIONER
On your first visit to a reflexologist, you will be asked questions relating to your general health and lifestyle. Leading a busy, stressful life can affect your overall health. While reflexology cannot take the stress out of your life, treatment can help you feel more relaxed.

You'll be asked to sit in a comfortable, reclining position that will allow the reflexologist to work on your feet. The soles of your feet will be examined and may be given a general massage with talcum powder to determine if there are tender and painful areas that need treatment. Treatment will then begin, with the reflexologist firmly but gently manipulating and stroking the feet, using both fingers and thumbs. It is not a painful process, but there may be momentary discomfort when the affected area is first stroked. Several points will be treated on both feet.

CAN I TREAT MYSELF?
It can be difficult to reach some of the points yourself, but you can use those you can reach to treat minor symptoms and conditions.

REFLEXOLOGY POINTS ON THE FEET

In many instances, there are matching points on both your feet. The points on your right foot are said to match the parts on the right side of your body; the ones on your left foot are said to correspond to those on your left side. There are several points, however, that can be found on only one foot, such as the ones for the heart, spleen, and gall bladder.

1 Brain/top of head
2 Sinuses/brain/top of head
3 Side of brain and head/neck
4 Pituitary gland
5 Spine
6 Neck/throat/thyroid gland
7 Parathyroid gland
8 Thyroid gland
9 Trachea
10 Eye
11 Eustachian tube
12 Ear
13 Shoulder
14 Lung

15 Heart
16 Solar plexus
17 Stomach
18 Pancreas
19 Kidney
20 Liver
21 Gall bladder
22 Spleen
23 Ascending colon
24 Descending colon
25 Small intestine
26 Bladder
27 Sciatic nerve

RIGHT FOOT

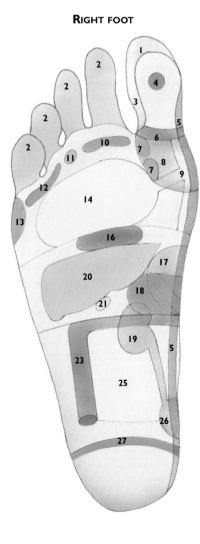

LEFT FOOT

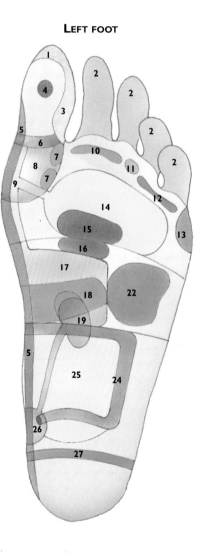

6

RELAXATION & VISUALIZATION

RELAXING AT WORK

It is important to release muscle tension at work—you'll both feel and perform better. Take a few minutes to do some stretching exercises, such as standing and stretching your arms to the ceiling, then to your toes, or stretching your arms behind your back. Even getting up and walking around for a few minutes can help.

HOW RELAXATION WORKS

True relaxation is not simply a case of stopping work for the evening. You have to take time to do it correctly. There are many health benefits to be had from relaxing properly, particularly in terms of relieving stress, which can lead to various health problems, such as digestive upsets, and even heart disease. Other conditions that relaxation techniques can help include:

- Pain
- Asthma
- Anxiety
- Nausea

Deep breathing is one way to reduce stress and is essential for relaxation. In fact, breathing exercises are an important part of the ancient traditions of yoga and meditation. Only a few minutes a day set aside for breathing exercises is all that's needed. ▶

BREATHING EXERCISES FOR RELAXING

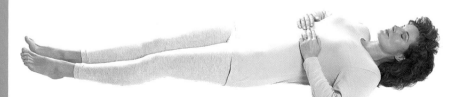

Chest breathing brings oxygen into the lungs quickly and is how we breathe when exercising or in a stressful situation. The exercise is a quick way to help you wake up in the morning and feel more alert when your energy is flagging.

Start by wearing comfortable clothes and removing any footwear. Lie on a comfortable firm surface, with your hands resting gently on your chest and close your eyes. Using the muscles in your chest, slowly breathe in and out. Your hands should rise when you breathe in and fall when you breathe out.

Diaphragm breathing is the natural way to breathe when you are relaxed. It brings more oxygen into the lungs than chest breathing does. Try it when you are stressed or tired, using your diaphragm to draw air in, rather than your chest.

Lying comfortably on the floor with your eyes closed, place your hands on your abdomen just below your rib cage and breathe in slowly. Feel your hands rising, then breathe out and feel them fall.

6

How visualization works

Visualization is a form of deep relaxation, in which a person tries to vividly imagine certain scenes. It is believed to be helpful for a variety of complaints, including panic and anxiety disorders, heart problems, and digestive disorders.

How do i do it?

Begin by sitting or lying comfortably somewhere that you know will be quiet for at least 15 minutes. As you get better at it you may be able to practice visualization anywhere, even in stressful situations. There are two types: external and internal visualization.

■ External visualization involves conjuring up images of things, for example, imagining that you are in a beautiful place or somewhere that you were particularly happy, such as an isolated sunny beach on vacation. Use your imagination to picture what is around you, including colors and textures. Try to imagine any smells that may be associated with the scene. Playing relaxing music can add to the atmosphere.

■ Internal visualization concentrates on imagining what is going on inside your own body to help it release muscle tension. Each group of muscles is tensed and then relaxed from head to toe. This is one of the best ways to reduce stress.

WHAT ELSE CAN I DO?

There are many other effective ways to relax, and what you do depends on your preferences.

■ Exercise, especially swimming, is a good form of relaxation for many people.

■ You can relax at home by making sure you unplug the phone and not attempting to do any household duties for an hour.

■ Gardening, reading, or soaking in a bathtub are all good ways to unwind.

INTERNAL VISUALIZATION EXERCISE

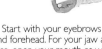

Progressive muscle relaxation releases stress. Lie comfortably on the floor with your eyes closed and take deep breaths from your diaphragm (see opposite). Tense each of the muscle groups for a count of 5 and then relax them.

Start with your eyebrows and forehead. For your jaw and face, open your mouth as wide as you can; then tense your neck and shoulder muscles. Lift your arms and tense them;

then tense your rib and stomach muscles. One at a time, raise your legs and tense them and your feet, then gently drop them. Now imagine yourself in a quiet place.

6

ADDRESSES

Use this page as a reminder of useful names and telephone numbers, and to record any information relevant to your family's medical history, which you should relay to a doctor or paramedic treating a member of your family. Make sure that anyone caring for your children knows where to find this information.

EMERGENCY SERVICES 911

ADDRESS

DOCTOR

DOCTOR

DOCTOR

DENTIST

LOCAL PHARMACY

POISON CONTROL CENTER   **HOSPITAL ER**

WORK NUMBERS

BABYSITTERS

DAYCARE CENTER

GRANDPARENTS

FRIENDS/NEIGHBORS

BLOOD TYPE

MEDICATION ALLERGIES

MEDICAL HISTORY

ACKNOWLEDGMENTS

l = left; r = right; b = bottom; t = top; c = centre

All illustrations by Mike Saunders except: p. 12-13, Rudi Vizi.
All photographs by Iain Bagwell except: pp. 22bl, 47, 81, 94bl, Andrew Sydenham; p. 81ltr, Laura Wickendon.

The publishers would like to thank the Chelsea Physic Garden for supplying the plants shown on pp 11, 13, 25, 32, 36l,

57b, 62, 68, 74, 76, 79, 82, 83, 87, 93; Gregory Bottley Lloyd for the minerals shown on pp 13r, 57t, 61, 64. and Patrick Carpenter for the mineral on p. 55br.

The publishers would also like to thank Design Assistants Philip Letsu and Michele Grigoletti Picture Editor Zilda Tandy DTP Editors Lesley Gilbert and Mary Pickles Editorial Co-ordinator Rebecca Clunes Research James Rankin Editorial Assistance John C Miles